The Communication Panacea

PEDIATRICS AND GENERAL SEMANTICS

Eva Berger
Isaac Berger

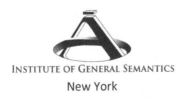

INSTITUTE OF GENERAL SEMANTICS

New York

Published by:

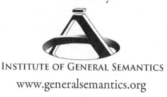

INSTITUTE OF GENERAL SEMANTICS
www.generalsemantics.org

First printing

Cover & Interior Book Design by Scribe Freelance

ISBN: 978-0-9860764-8-0

Published in the United States of America

Library of Congress Cataloging-in-Publication Data

Berger, Eva, Dr., author.
 The communication panacea : pediatrics and general semantics / Eva Berger, Isaac Berger.
  p. ; cm. -- (New non-Aristotelian library series)
 Includes bibliographical references and index.
 ISBN 978-0-9860764-8-0 (pbk. : alk. paper)
 I. Berger, Isaac, 1938- , author. II. Institute of General Semantics, publisher. III. Title. IV. Series: New non-Aristotelian library series.
 [DNLM: 1. Pediatrics. 2. Semantics. 3. Communication. 4. Physician-Patient Relations. WS 100]
 R727.3
 610.69'6--dc23
                    2014041410

For Zlate

CONTENTS

———

FOREWORD

———■———

I N 1963, WHILE living in Chicago for his residency with his wife
Zlate and one year old daughter Eva (his co-author of this book),
Zlate told Isaac that her sister would be coming for a short visit
from Mexico. In a solemn tone, she asked him to sit down with her in
the living room, as she needed to talk to him. Not knowing what to
expect and getting ready for some dramatic news, he heard from his
wife for the first time that her sister was diabetic. She was diagnosed
years before but had been prohibited by her mother to tell anyone, as
was everyone else in the house. Zlate had been told not to tell Isaac,
in spite of the fact that he was a physician, for fear that the news
would prompt him to leave her. And the sister herself was not
allowed to mention it because if she did, nobody would want to
marry her. But there was no choice now. Mina would be arriving in a
few weeks with her medicine and her syringes, so there would be no
way of hiding the disease from him and, besides, he was a doctor and
he needed to know so that he could help if there were any problems.

Mina was diagnosed with Type 1 diabetes (formerly called
juvenile-onset or insulin-dependent diabetes) at the age of 12 at a
time when treatment was much more complex and the chances of
surviving beyond a certain age were much slimmer than today. The
diagnosis was thus a terrifying label that put great psychological
pressure on children in addition to the difficulties that came with the
measuring of sugar levels, injecting insulin a few times a day, and
abstaining from eating many of the foods loved by children. And
there was the cultural context, too: A Jewish family of European
immigrants to Mexico for whom marriage was very important.

Mina died at the age of 30, survived by her loving sisters, her husband and her daughter.

Diagnoses are the names doctors give to combinations of symptoms. They are the labels given to illnesses, guiding much more than just treatments and decisions about medication. Depending on the social and cultural norms, as well as a patient's personal psychology, an illness, its diagnosis, can mean, in addition to the objective physical symptoms of the disease, the degradation of a person's identity and a permanent stigma. Diagnoses can be iatrogenic labels. In other words, they may intensify stress, define incapacity, impose inactivity, and focus on uncertainty which leads to the loss of autonomy for self-definition. They often isolate people in their role as patients, separating them from the normal and healthy, and requiring submission to the authority of doctors and nurses.

Awareness of the language of medicine and its implications on health care, including diagnoses, especially in the context of pediatrics, is at the heart of this book and it brings together the professional fields of its authors. Isaac is a retired pediatrician with over 50 years of experience and Eva, his daughter, is a professor of Communication.

At some point it became clear to us that our conversations throughout the years always revolved around the semantic environment of medicine and that we shared our passion for thinking of ways to make that environment as pollution free as possible. The book was born at the Eureka moment when we realized that the principles of General Semantics provide the most coherent framework for thinking about the subject, and that without being aware of the specific principles during his career, Isaac had intuitively acted based on them in the treatment of his patients.

We would like to acknowledge a number of people whose help and support made this book possible. First we would like to thank

Corey Anton, General Editor of the New Non-Aristotelian Library; Marty Levinson, President of the Board of Trustees of the Institute of General Semantics; and Lance Strate, Professor of Communication and Media Studies at Fordham University and old friend.

We would also like to thank Yuval, Eva's husband for his patience, support and encouragement as well as his smart criticism, his suggestions and his love. We thank Etai and Jonathan, Eva's sons and Isaac's grandsons, for so naturally talking to their mother for months with the back of a laptop covering half of her face. And we thank Zlate, Isaac's wife and Eva's mom, for her enthusiastic participation in all of our conversations and her aid to Isaac in recalling the stories of his patients. We dedicate the book to her.

Finally, Isaac wishes to express his gratitude to all of his patients and their parents throughout the years for their lessons of courage, of gratitude and of love.

INTRODUCTION

———■———

*Doctors will have more lives to answer for in the next
world than even we generals.*

—Napoleon Bonaparte

THE PAST 50 YEARS or so have been characterized by an increasing dissatisfaction with the relationships between doctors and patients. To paraphrase Wildavsky (1977), people seem to be doing better but they are feeling worse.

Developments in medicine, along with improved diet and public health measures have reduced deaths from infection and extended life. Doctors are saving people who would have died only a generation ago. But alongside the scientific progress and new cures available, clinical practice keeps getting increasingly impersonal, commercialized and technological. Patients are more doubtful about how genuine doctors' concern for them are as people, and doctors feel that patients are becoming less compliant and are more challenging to their authority.

The dissatisfaction stems, at least in part, from patients' conception of the historical ideal of the personal or family physician that had trusting and long-term relationships with their patients. Doctors still see patients, of course, and some even have long term relationships with them, especially in the realm of primary care. But the environment in which these encounters take place has changed. The relationships take place now in impersonal settings such as hospitals, emergency rooms or clinics and they are usually hurried, mediated by technology, and paid for by third parties.

The cultural conception of doctors at around the end of the nineteenth century was, as Shorter (1991) explains, of wise and observant men, as can be learned from art of the era such as Luke Fildes' 1891 painting, *The Doctor*. They relied less on instruments and more on compassion and good judgment and they were almost exclusively male.

By 1920, public health measures had reduced the incidence and in some cases entirely eliminated many diseases such as smallpox, yellow fever, cholera or typhus, and over the course of the twentieth century, patients began to visit doctors more often for less serious conditions such as colds or skin problems. But in spite of the increased scientific knowledge, some infectious diseases such as tuberculosis, diphtheria or scarlet fever remained lethal until the 1940's and 50's.

The modern doctor-patient relationship developed against this background. It was very common for doctors to make house calls to patients suffering of these diseases, and the house calls entailed a careful physical examination. Patients did not expect to be cured, but they did expect to be cared for and comforted, which was believed to have healing powers in itself.

These encounters were, however, not entirely tension-free, as even then the doctor's livelihood depended on the fees paid for his services, so he had to satisfy the expectations of his patients which wasn't always an easy task. As George Bernard Shaw put it in *The Doctor's Dilemma* (1911):

> The doctor who has to live by pleasing his patients in competition with everybody, who has walked the hospitals, scraped through the examinations and bought a brass plate, soon finds himself prescribing water to teetotalers and brandy or champagne jelly to

drunkards; beefsteaks and stout in one house, and uric acid free vegetarian diet over the way. (p.1xxxi)

To this tension between the self-interest of the physician and the best interests of the patient, a new one was added between the increasingly technological and biomedical focus on disease and the care of the patient.

Major diagnostic technologies developed such as the microscope, X-rays, the sphygmomanometer (to measure blood pressure), and electrocardiographs among others. These transformed the measurement as well as the perception of disease and paradoxically, as the technologies made their way into offices of family doctors and hospitals, the personal relationship between physicians and patients began to weaken. As medicine became increasingly scientific, it also became more impersonal, mechanistic and remote. The emphasis moved from patients to disease, doctors began to be more and more specialized, and the availability of family doctors and primary care physicians who knew their patients as a whole person and who had lasting relationships with them decreased. As the humanist physician Sir William Osler explained (as quoted by Cushing, 1925), the new scientific medicine of diagnostic precision was endangering the old medicine of care and compassion. Osler advised doctors to stay away from what he called "the many useless drugs" and to stay focused on the patient as a person. "The good physician," he said, "treats the disease, but the great physician treats the patient." And along the same lines, Harvard Professor of Medicine Francis W. Peabody (1927), pointed out that patients in advanced university hospitals were sometimes passed from one specialist to another, submitted to multiple tests, and treated for unimportant conditions. He added that with the exception of the relationship that one may have with a member of one's family, or with the priest, there is no human bond like the one between physician and patient (or the patient's family). Nevertheless, these bonds were constantly weakened and the house calls, which had allowed physicians to understand patients in the context of their families, began to disappear. Among other reasons for their disappearance was doctors' increasing realization that house calls were keeping their income down because they limited the number of patients they could see in a day.

Developments in non-medical technologies were affecting the process of distancing between physicians and patients, too. For example, with the growth of the suburbs and the use of cars, doctors' practices started to move beyond their own communities. The growth of private insurance payments and the introduction of Medicare and Medicaid in 1972 generated new sources of income and introduced another impersonal actor that undercut the personal qualities of traditional fee-for-service medicine. This turned patients more apprehensive of doctors who were suspected as being motivated by greed. And revelations in the media about the abuse of human subjects in medical research further shook the public's faith in physicians. The insistence on informed consent and the right to refuse treatment marked an important shift in the power and center of focus of decision-making that was moving from the physician to the autonomous patient. The reign of benevolent paternalism was coming to an end.

But one of the key forces in the downfall of the modern doctor-patient relationship was the corporate transformation of American medicine that began in the 1980s. Independent professional doctors became employees of hospitals, insurance companies and health care corporations. And pharmaceutical companies played an important role, too, as they found themselves increasingly under financial pressures to find new diseases among healthy people, and to satisfy the security analysts. They began to lobby for the reclassification of conditions by, for example, constantly moving the line that marks what is regarded as normal blood pressure so that someone who was once in the upper part of the range and defined as "normotensive" is now "pre-hypertensive," even if there are no symptoms to justify this. This new definition of normal blood pressure allows pharmaceutical companies, of course, to adjust and refine their sales to get doctors to overprescribe. No wonder the Greek term "pharmakon" is ambiguous, and it can mean both "cure" and "poison."

In short, medicine has become more and more dominated by bureaucratic authority and motivated by commercial gain; doctors are seeing more and more patients per day, and it has become more and more difficult for them to advocate for their patients. And this has obviously led to patient dissatisfaction but also to growing rates of doctor burnout and depression.

As a response to this state of affairs, a host of theories and movements aimed at humanizing the relationship between doctors and patients and improving communication between them have been developed. These include the fields of Bioethics, the Medical Humanities, Narrative Medicine, Spirituality in Medicine, Patient-Centered Care, and Health Communication.

Scholars in the field of Health Communication study physician-patient communication from a variety of perspectives and approaches. Over the past three decades, numerous models of the physician-patient relationship have been developed and advocated with varying degrees of enthusiasm (e.g., Emanuel & Emanuel, 1992; Leopold, Cooper, & Clancy, 1996). Many of the models were developed and offered as alternatives to paternalistic approaches to the physician-patient relationship (Emanuel & Emanuel, 1992). Other models were influenced by ideas consistent with bio-psycho-social approaches to health care. But as Cegala and Street (2009) explain, much remains to be done with respect to providing meaningful, theoretical accounts of processes affecting communication and outcomes, as well as creating measures that integrate behavioral and perceptual features of communication.

This book's purpose is to make a contribution in that direction on the basis of the field called General Semantics that allows us to understand medicine as a semantic environment and not only as a profession or as a service.

General semantics is a practical discipline that applies modern scientific thinking to the solution of personal and professional problems. The application of its principles allows for clearer thinking, more effective and accurate communication and interactions, as well as more appropriate responses to what happens. It helps avoid prejudice, stereotyping, and generalizations and to understand and evaluate the underlying assumptions of other people's assumptions as well as one's own. And to modify them based on observation.

If adopted, the principles of General Semantics lead, generally, to greater sanity in life. Thus, we find them to be the panacea or medicine to cure or at least alleviate the symptoms of the illnesses of modern day medicine and to reduce the number of cases afflicted with what we shall later call "Semantic Iatrogenic Disease."

Chapter 1 of the book is devoted to the idea of "semantic iatrogenesis" – harm inflicted by physicians through doctor-talk and communication patterns that intensify and even induce illness. After defining what we mean by semantic iatrogenesis we introduce the concept of a semantic environment, and explain in general terms, the usefulness of General Semantics in keeping the medical semantic environment clean and free of sematic pollution.

Chapter 2 of the book is devoted to the specific semantic environment of pediatrics. We encourage doctors and patients to look at pediatrics not only as a medical specialty, but as a special semantic environment due to its triadic nature and the ages of the patients.

In Chapter 3 we go into the specific tools that General Semantics provides pediatricians to fight Semantic Iatrogenic Disease, beginning with an understanding of the difference and connections between the context and the content of semantic environments: both the physical and emotional aspects of the medical encounter, doctors diagnoses and definitions of illness, as well as the metaphors employed throughout history when thinking of pediatrics – pediatrics as exploration and pediatrics as veterinary medicine.

After establishing the context and explaining our central terminology, in Part II of the book we move on to illustrate sematic iatrogenesis as well as the use of General Semantics to counter it. Beginning with a distinction between curing, healing and doctoring, in Chapter 4 we tell the stories of eight of the patients of the medical doctor among us and parallel to the relatively new term of Personalized Genetic Medicine, we propose the development and practice of what we call "Personalized Semantic Medicine."

We tell of Ami and the triumph of his metaphor of "having sickness" over the common metaphor of "being sick." Hassan's story is one about Isaac's refusal to be governed by the Chief of Pediatrics' definitions and policies, for the good of the patient. Dalia's mom's story revolves around the need for doctors to ask good questions, and the next story tells of the lesson a patient taught Isaac about the dangers of mystifying patients and the importance of avoiding role fixation. At the center of the following story is Dani who was having recurring nightmares that sent the parents into a self-reflexive spiral. And the next story is all about time-binding – when patients stick around and their pediatrician becomes their own children's pediatrician. The story about the quintuplets born at Isaac's hospital is about children's individuality and the need for indexing. And Jack's story is about the difficulty of inferring experience from behavior.

Chapter 5 discusses the latest trends in medicine stemming from policy and economics as well as from the technological innovations of the past few years and illustrates how the problems encountered by Isaac have been further exasperated, bringing us to the brink of a semantic iatrogenic epidemic, creating the need for doctors who are general semanticists and for a new kind of doctoring that we call Subversive Doctoring.

Our conclusion chapter summarizes the thesis presented throughout the book that the principles of General Semantics provide a most useful tool for more effective communication in the medical environment; that General Semantics is the panacea that can act as both remedy and preventive medicine against Semantic Iatrogenic Disease. In this final chapter we also suggest that not only doctors need to be subversive but so must patients whose role is also key in making the semantic environment pollution free. And that the way to achieve this is by replacing the metaphor of medicine as war with that of medicine as art.

PART I

CHAPTER 1
Semantic Iatrogenesis

———■———

A doctor is the conjunction of a white coat,
a stethoscope, and a jargon.

—Adolfo Bioy Casares

ILANA HAD BEEN experiencing excruciating pain in her elbow for almost a year. She had gotten a few shots, had taken part in an experimental study, and nothing seemed to work. At the dinner table one night, she told us the story of her latest visit to the doctor. He never examined her. He just wanted to talk to her. So she sat across the desk from him telling him of how it was getting harder and harder to do even the most daily chores. He never picked his eyes up from the computer screen and still typing, he said: "You are simply hitting your backhand wrong."

He must have noticed the word "tennis" somewhere in Ilana's Electronic Health Record, and purely on its basis diagnosed what was wrong with her elbow – and her game. It was, of course, tennis elbow. But had the doctor taken a moment to really listen to Ilana, he would have found out that she was a professional tennis player for about 20 years, Israel's champ five years in a row, and famous for her killer backhand. He would have also found out that she was now a coach, that the pain was interfering with her livelihood, with her income, and that she was worried about the future.

Ilana experienced first-hand the implications of an increasingly technological and bureaucratic health system in Israel. She was a victim of the EHR, of the 8-minute appointment, and of the overscheduled doctor. The computer screens and EHR's that doctors look at while talking to us these days is only one of the newest in a series of technologies that have mediated between doctors and patients throughout history. Each new medical technology, each new screen in the clinic or the hospital, has brought us closer to an apparently accurate representation of our bodies, in sickness and in health, or at least to the illusion thereof. As Reiser (1978) explains:

> [The invention of the stethoscope] helped to create the objective physician, who could move away from involvement with the patient's experiences and sensations, to a more detached relation, less with the patient but more with the sounds from within the body. Undistracted by the motives and beliefs of the patient, the auscultator could make a diagnosis from sounds that he alone heard emanating from body organs, sounds that he believed to be objective, bias-free representations of the disease process. (p. 38)

This detachment and illusion of objectivity became even truer with visual medical imaging technologies that enable the physician to further disregard the patient's motives and feelings, or worse, regard them as "wrong" and the picture as "true." With these technologies the detachment from patients increased and the art of listening began to falter. Instead of performing as aids in the process of diagnosis, the stethoscope, X-rays, the electrocardiograph, ultrasound, MRIs, and other technologies almost entirely replaced conversation.

Patients, too, have come to rely completely on tests. They demand them; they feel cheated when not referred to have them done; and they sue for malpractice when doctors fail to accurately interpret them. This, in turn, creates an atmosphere in which medical competence is defined by the quantity and variety of technologies brought to bear on the disease.

In this mediated reality--where pathologists and radiologists interpret the meaning of technical information and have no connection whatsoever with the patient, only with tissue and photographs--the message, as Postman (1992) put it, is that "medicine is about disease, not the patient. What the patient knows is untrustworthy; what the machine knows is reliable" (p.100). This is iatrogenesis at its clearest.

Iatrogenesis is generally defined as harm inflicted by doctors. And "semantic iatrogenesis," as we will suggest, is the harm done to patients that results from what doctors say and how they react, and from their finding patients' descriptions of what they are feeling and experiencing less reliable than the images of their organs on a screen.

Semantic iatrogenesis is, in other words, harm inflicted by doctors' use of language. But in spite of doctors' language being a central focal point of the field of Health Communication, what we mean by it here is not only doctors' use of medical jargon.

The use of professional jargon that sounds like a foreign language to patients is, indeed, the source of some of the problems in doctor-patient communication. Medical jargon, as in other professions, is the language by which practitioners in different areas conduct their businesses and endeavors and through which they differentiate themselves from others and claim their status. As Castro, et al. (2007) explain, there may be several reasons for why physicians employ jargon with patients. Starting in medical school, doctors are trained in a context known as the "culture of medicine," that values efficient transmission of highly technical information and relies on a distinct language to achieve this goal. They use this language either because they overestimate their patients' understanding of their terminology or because through it, they assert their professionalism. And the authors even consider the possibility that they use this specialized language to empower patients by exposing them to concepts and terms relevant to the self-management of their illness. Whichever the reason, the dangers in the use of professional jargon are bigger in medicine than in other professions as in medicine, sometimes life itself is at stake. Confused by unclear instructions and complex medical phrases, patients are more likely to skip necessary medical tests or fail to properly take their medications. And the issue has become more urgent with advances in medicine that have made treatment decisions more complex. But, in any case, the problem of semantic iatrogenesis is much deeper than just the use of jargon.

In *The Normal and the Pathological,* George Canguilhem (1989) analyzes the radically new way in which health and disease were defined in the early 19th-century, showing that the emerging categories of the normal and the pathological were far from being objective scientific concepts. He talks about how the epistemological foundations of medicine were intertwined with political, economic, and technological imperatives, and as a medical relativist, he explains that diseases are not absolute entities and do not exist as such in nature, and that the definition of what is normal and what pathological depends on the circumstances in which they are observed. In this context, he speaks of the term iatrogenesis--or harm caused by the healer ("iatros," the Greek word for "physician" and "genesis" meaning "origin")--and wonders why it was not until the 1950s that the idea received the attention it deserved.

As Nassim Nicholas Taleb (2012) explains, medicine has known about iatrogenesis since at least the fourth century B.C. The principle of "Primum non nocere" ("first do no harm") is attributed to Hippocrates and integrated in the Hippocratic Oath taken by every doctor on his or her commencement day. Yet in spite of its recitations through the ages, the term "iatrogenesis" only appeared in frequent use a few decades ago.

Taleb (2012) claims that, until penicillin, medicine had a largely negative balance sheet and going to the doctor increased people's chance of death. But he adds that it is telling that iatrogenesis increased over time, along with knowledge, and peaked late in the nineteenth century: it was "scientific progress," the birth of the clinic and its substitution for home remedies that caused death rates to shoot up, mostly from what was then called "hospital fever." He provides some statistics and says that medical error still currently kills between three and ten times as many people as car accidents in the United States and that harm from doctors—not including risks from hospital germs—accounts for more deaths than any single cancer.

Ivan Illich (1976) goes even farther and argues that the medical establishment has become a major threat to health, and that the disabling impact of the professional control over medicine has reached the proportions of an epidemic. The name he gives to the epidemic is "iatrogenesis" and he describes three kinds of iatrogenesis: clinical, social and cultural.

Clinical iatrogenesis includes all of the clinically verifiable, specific health-denying or disease-making effects of specific medical interventions, pathologies increased through the practice of medicine. Clinical iatrogenic disease comprises all clinical conditions for which remedies, doctors, or hospitals are the pathogens, or "sickening" agents. They are a sort of therapeutic side-effects. According to Illich these are as old as medicine itself, and have always been a subject of medical studies. And he divides clinical iatrogenesis into four categories: Negligence or professional callousness; accidents, human error or systems break down; specific accepted risks--the diseases of medical progress inevitably connected with the administration of certain cures or diagnostic tools; and finally, of course, the damage that results from doctors' attempts to protect themselves against malpractice suits.

The second kind of iatrogenesis is social iatrogenesis which is expressed in various symptoms of social over-medicalization that amount to what Illich calls "the expropriation of health." He includes here all impairments to health that are due to socio-economic transformations stemming from the institutional shape of health care. In other words, what he is concerned with here are the iatrogenic effects of the social structure, social behavior, and social rituals built around the application of medical technology to people who are supposedly sick and to their environment. And he provides an example: The medicalization of family structure that happens when dying at home becomes socially inconceivable, when aging at home becomes increasingly more painful rather than more beautiful, thanks to our progress in scientific knowledge and technology. In other words, social iatrogenesis takes place when the environment loses the conditions that provide individuals, families, and neighborhoods with control over their own internal states and over their milieu.

The third kind of iatrogenesis is cultural and it consists of the disappearance of healthy responses to suffering and death. It occurs when people accept and come to expect health management designed on the engineering model, and when they think of health as a commodity and talk about "better health" or, as Illich puts it:

> Professionally organized medicine has come to function as a domineering moral enterprise that advertises industrial expansion as a war against all suffering. It has thereby undermined the ability of individuals to face their reality, to express their own values, and to accept inevitable and often irremediable

pain and impairment, decline and death. (p. 51)

These three categories seem to cover most of the damages inflicted by physicians, but one area that Illich and others neglect to discuss is the damage caused by doctors that stems from their use of language.

Some sources, such as those within the specific practice of psychiatry where one of the central tools is language, devote some attention to the potential harm that using the wrong words may cause. Boisvert et al. (2002) for example, discuss the power of certain metaphors on patients' self-perception; or certain labels or definitions as they are included in the DSM (*Diagnostic and Statistical Manual of Mental Disorders* published by the American Psychiatric Association) as self-fulfilling prophecies. It is also telling, we believe, that the authors themselves call patients "clients." But this kind of medical literature is specific and sporadic and does not amount to a coherent theory. Thus, it is our belief that a new category is necessary in the description and analysis of physician inflicted harm. In addition to clinical, social and cultural iatrogenesis, we need to study what may be called "semantic iatrogenesis" – harm inflicted by physicians through doctor-talk and communication patterns that intensify and even induce illness.

Illich (1976) claims that medical bureaucracy creates ill-health by increasing stress, by multiplying dependence, and by lowering the levels of tolerance for discomfort or pain. But he also adds, without developing it any further, that "social iatrogenesis is at work when the language in which people could experience their bodies is turned into bureaucratic gobbledegook" (p.16).

Anyone who has come in contact with doctors, nurses and modern complex health systems generally has encountered examples of this "bureaucratic gobbledegook." From the moment doctors were transformed from artisans exercising a skill on individuals they knew personally, into technicians applying scientific rules to classes of patients, the language used to describe processes, and especially problems within processes, changed. What had formerly been considered an abuse of confidence or a moral fault began to be rationalized into "the occasional breakdown of equipment." In technology rich hospitals, negligence became "random human error" or "system breakdown," callousness became "scientific detachment," and incompetence became "a lack of specialized equipment." The depersonalization of diagnosis and care brought about a new vocabulary to describe malpractice: the language of ethics was replaced by the language of technology and technique.

In a world lead by the language of bureaucracy--of technology and technique--when we get sick we don't meet in the eyes of the doctor a reflection or recognition of our personal suffering. Instead, we encounter the gaze of a medical accountant of sorts, engaged in input and output calculations. Our illness is taken away from us and turned into the stuff of an institutional enterprise or the basis for research. Our condition is interpreted according to a set of abstract rules in a language we cannot understand. If doctors consider it necessary to gain our cooperation, they will tell us of the "thing" they are setting out to "combat." Language is taken over by doctors and we are deprived of meaningful words to describe our anguish, which leads to what general semanticists call "mystification."

And this doesn't happen only when we are sick. Being a responsible person in the world of medical bureaucracy means periodically going for "check-ups." As Illich (1976) points out,

> People keep up with the Joneses by emulating their "check-ups." People are turned into patients without being sick. The medicalization of prevention...tends

to transform personal responsibility for my future
into my management by some agency. (p. 35)

The agents make patients increasingly dependent on the special
language of their elite profession, turning disease into an instrument
of class domination. Patients are put in their place as subjects who do
not speak the language of their master.

In other words, medicine is a moral enterprise and, as such, it
defines what is normal or abnormal. It has the power to label one
complaint a legitimate ailment and to refuse recognition of another,
as well as to declare someone sick without them even knowing that
they are. It has the authority to label one pain as "imagined" or
"psychosomatic," and even to call one death "suicide" but not
another. Doctors decide what a symptom is and who is sick. And
every time they make a new diagnosis, they appropriate the power of
definition and create a new group of outsiders.

"Mystification" and "definition" are two of the terms at the
center of the field of study called General Semantics. At the basis of
General Semantics is the idea that humans have a tendency to misuse
language – what Postman (1976) calls "Crazy Talk" and "Stupid
Talk"--and that this leads to dysfunctional communication--what
Johnson (1946) calls "quandaries." In his book under the same title –
Crazy Talk, Stupid Talk – Postman says: "Physicians are notoriously
guilty of both mystifying and terrifying patients by using polysyllabic
technical terms to denote commonplace and easily curable disorders."
And, he continues:

> In fact, within the past few years, there has grown up
> a field known as iatrogenics...Though the term itself
> is unnecessarily mysterious, the idea of having a field
> within a field to monitor the harmful consequences
> of verbal mystification is, in my opinion, a splendid

one, and I would urge its replication in every field. (p. 228)

As it turns out, the idea of iatrogenesis has now been applied, by extension, to the side effects of policy makers or academics, and one can now read about how, for example, "the credit crisis was the result of rampant iatrogenesis." However, in spite of Postman's enthusiasm, it turns out as well that in medicine – the field from which the concept originated – most of the emphasis has been placed, as previously discussed, on clinical iatrogenesis, and much less on the harmful consequences of doctors' language.

And so, we take on Postman's challenge here and place at the center of our thesis the idea that misuses of language are--in the area of health care and medicine--a major source of iatrogenesis, thus the term "semantic iatrogenesis."

It is our hope, of course, that doctors and health professionals will benefit from our ideas here. But patients may benefit from them, too. There isn't much patients, as individuals, can do to avoid or fight the other three kinds of iatrogenesis. But as partners in conversation with doctors, patients can take responsibility for their health, beginning with an awareness of how the medical profession talks, and thus thinks and operates. This may, as Illich (1976) suggests,

> ...lead to an environment of self-reliance, autonomy, and dignity. [An] environment [that] brings out an autonomous personal and responsible coping ability. (p. 5)

Illich uses the word environment here in its most general sense. But in order to understand how language and its misuse can bring about illness or delay healing or how semantic iatrogenesis works, it is important to qualify the word "environment" and speak, as general semanticists do, of a semantic environment. "We often speak about the influence of heredity," says Korzybski (1958), and he adds, "...but much less do we analyse what influence environment, and particularly the verbal environment, has upon us" (p. 270).

A semantic environment is defined by Postman (1969) as "any human situation in which language plays a critical role" (p.15). He goes on to explain that the constituents of an environment are people, their purposes, and the language they use to help them achieve those purposes. And that because there are so many human purposes, there are many different kinds of semantic environments. Politics is a semantic environment; science and commerce are semantic environments. And, of course, medicine is a semantic environment.

It is interesting to point out that the metaphors used by Postman to explain what a semantic environment is, come from the realm of both ecology and health. "A healthy semantic environment" he says, "is one in which language effectively serves the purposes of the particular context in which it is used" (pp. 15-16). Thus, if the language used in the medical context serves the purpose of healing it is a healthy semantic environment. And the opposite of this is true as well. When language obscures from people, what they are doing and why, Postman adds, "the semantic environment is polluted, and stops serving the purposes it is supposed to serve" (p. 16). In such cases, the environment "sickens and becomes useless" (p. 14). In the case of medical environments, the sickening pollution is what we call here "semantic iatrogenesis."

It is possible to keep pollution away and to keep the medical semantic environment healthy. In order to do so, a deep understanding and application of the central concepts of General Semantics such as consciousness of abstracting, semantic reactions, extensional orientation, etc. are necessary. And, as we explain in the next chapter, nowhere is this more critical than in the semantic sub-environment of pediatrics.

CHAPTER 2
The Semantic Environment of Pediatrics

———■———

Children are the living messages we send
to a time we will not see
—Neil Postman

THE ILLNESS OF A child requires the re-organization not only of the parent's life-story but of the child's life-story in the minds of parents, too. The loss of the previously taken-for-granted continuity of life in chronically ill people is regarded as especially tragic in the case of children. Pediatrics presents a special challenge. As Kleinman and Seeman (2000) explain, the experience of illness is not bounded by the bodies or consciousness of those who are ill. It reaches out to encompass a household, a family, or a social network. And this is especially true when the patient is a child.

Streisand and Tercyak (2004) explain that all parents are challenged with the task of promoting normal, healthy development in their children. This includes promoting not only physical growth and maturation, but social, emotional, and intellectual development as well. For parents of children with a chronic illness, these challenges are intensified, because helping children to achieve their developmental milestones must occur within the parameters of the child's medical adversity. At times, childhood illness interrupts or delays normal development. This can result in a widening gap between the resources, skills, and achievements of children with illness relative to their healthy peers, thereby further increasing the worries, stresses, and burdens faced by their parents.

Chronic illness in children creates very unique circumstances for the children themselves and for their parents. Pediatric illness is an acutely stressful event, and the stress associated with it can profoundly impact long-term outcomes.

The impact that the illness has on the parent is thought to play a role in how the child adapts to the medical adversity. For example, anxiety on the part of the parent can affect the child's recovery process. Thus, it is imperative that clinical practice promotes an enhanced quality of life among children, parents, and their family members.

There is a longstanding tradition of health professionals that from the early 20th century, wrote about this topic. Arnold Gesell (1940), who was both a psychologist and physician, wrote and lectured about psychological principles in pediatric medicine, and the relationship between child behavior and development. And pediatrician Benjamin Spock's book *Baby and Child Care* (2004) was published for the first time in 1946. This book would later go on to sell more than 50 million copies worldwide, and was translated into more than 30 languages. Spock's message of patience, tolerance, and love for children influenced the attitudes and practices of generations of parents throughout the world. However, these and other popular resources primarily concentrated on physically healthy children; far less was known about parenting in the face of medical adversity.

In the early 1960s, Green and Solnit (1964) wrote about "vulnerable child syndrome." At its basis, this syndrome was about the altered relationship between parent and child when the child experienced an acute illness. The authors recognized that ill children would often be viewed by their parents as being almost fragile. They hypothesized that this parental view would lead to child maladjustment over time.

In the latter part of the 20th century, theoretical models began to emerge that focused on factors affecting psychosocial adjustment among children with chronic conditions, and emphasized the importance of parental adjustment and other familial and social factors in promoting child behavioral functioning under adverse medical circumstances (Wallander et al., 1989).

Various important themes assess the social, behavioral and psychological implications of illness in children. One of the most important ones is what is known as "pediatric parenting stress," which sources include negotiating complex health care systems and learning to communicate with providers around the jargon of the child's disease, among others.

Parents are children's most important health resource, helping them to manage the illness, while continuously bringing the child's medical needs to the attention of health care providers. Parents are an integral component of the identification and management of behavioral concerns, and the nature and quality of their communications with professionals about such problems often determine if and when intervention services are offered (Garrison et al., 1992; Horwitz et al., 1998).

The developmental phase of the child also affects the impact of the illness. As Streisand and Tercyak (2004) explain, physical illness during infancy significantly impacts both the infant and the parent. While parents of children of all ages have an innate desire to protect their children, parents of infants may also feel at fault for "causing" the infant's difficulties (perhaps through passing on inherited diseases), or feel incapable of managing their child's care. Some may even come to question their competency as parents in general.

Similar to infants, toddlers and preschoolers, or children aged 18 months through 5 years, are largely dependent on their parents or care-givers. But the challenges to parenting here are more related to helping children understand their illness, and helping them to co-operate with treatment. Because of their use of "magical thinking," children may come to believe they are to blame for the illness or painful medical regimens, and parents may feel at a loss over how to explain the need for various procedures to them. Also, development of self-control (so important in preschoolers) can also be affected by illness as children are precluded from making choices, and parents are reluctant to set appropriate limits on behavior.

For school-aged children (6-11 years), accomplishing developmental tasks is largely affected by interactions with peers, with children at this age using social comparison to help them judge their competencies in various domains of life. Disruption in normal routines due to illness can limit children's opportunities for social interactions. This may hamper the personal growth typically gained from peer interaction.

Perhaps the largest body of literature related to children's health and their development focuses on the transition to adolescence (ages 12-18 years). Many challenges occur at this phase, including identity formation, struggling with body image issues, and the move towards independence. These tasks may be particularly challenging for the adolescent with an illness. The task of independence poses particular challenges for parents of children who are ill. Just when parents are beginning to relinquish some responsibilities for the adolescent, an illness can easily overwhelm and alter this situation, necessitating parents once again to become intimately involved in every aspect of the teenager's life. This causes difficulties for the adolescent, the parent, and also the parent-adolescent relationship.

All of this is obvious to us these days. But it wasn't always so. Pediatrics is a relatively young medical specialty. As Postman (1982) explains, childhood is a social artifact as much as it is a biological category. As a social principle and a psychological condition it emerged around the sixteenth century. Up until then, children were not regarded as significantly different from adults. There were no special institutions to nurture them, no books on childrearing, and they were regarded primarily as economic utilities.

Childhood as we understand it today was an outgrowth of literacy. Children began to be separated from adults to be taught how to read. Ever since (or at least until the advent of television, according to Postman), human development began to be viewed as a series of stages, with childhood as a bridge between infancy and adulthood.

With the separation of children from adults, children's literature appeared, children's clothing was distinguished from that of adults', toys and games were invented, and eventually, the medical specialization of pediatrics.

The history of pediatrics spans less than two centuries. Prior to the development of pediatrics, the medical needs of infants and children were provided by families, friends, and midwives; physicians rarely contributed to the health of this population.

According to Connolly (2005), the first medical lectures on the diseases of childhood were offered in 1860 by physician Abraham Jacobi, considered by most to be founder of modern pediatrics. Until the Civil War, pediatrics was considered part of obstetrics in the United States. Before Jacobi, specialties centered on a particular organ or technology and not on an age-group. Jacobi felt that pediatrics should have a broader, more conceptual, focus. He believed that pediatricians should concern themselves with child health in general and not only on disease. He thought pediatricians should be involved in infant feeding, child hygiene, and disease prevention in healthy children. And he argued that "The pediatrician could also use his talents to facilitate the Americanization of immigrants." In short, the focus of Jacobi's model for pediatrics was well beyond specific diseases. It involved disease prevention in healthy children, educating parents about child rearing, and social activism for children's rights.

In 1880, Jacobi and a few other doctors founded the American Medical Association's section on the Diseases of Children. And in 1888 a new organization, the American Pediatric Society, helped to solidify pediatrics as a distinct branch of medicine. In other words, with the development of pediatrics, a new medical semantic environment (or, in Postman's terms--sub-environment) was created.

The sub-environment of pediatrics is quite different from the others, not only because of the illnesses treated or the specialty required, but also (and primarily) because of the age of the patients and the presence of a parent or guardian in the medical encounter. This makes for a semantic environment characterized not by dyadic interactions between adults (doctor-patient interactions) but on the doctor-parent-child triad, leading to very different purposes and relationships, and requiring a deep understanding of context, and an especially heightened semantic flexibility, as the level of abstraction required to make diagnoses clear, is different for parents and for children. And even with children, the level of abstraction needs to be adjusted based on the age of the child.

The evaluation of what language is appropriate in the medical treatment of children proceeds from an assessment of the specific purpose of pediatrics, and not from the general notion of the purpose of medicine-- as reflected from the Hippocratic Oath. The different participants in the pediatric semantic environment can have very different assessments of the situation. In the end, all the participants' objective is healing, of course, but parents of sick children may also need help with coping with the illness themselves, with helping their children understand and cope, with handling siblings at home, and addressing their feelings of guilt, etc. The pediatrician may be focused on curing the disease, but the patients may, at different points in time, require help with the labels attached to them by peers at school.

As mentioned earlier, physician-patient communication has been studied from various perspectives. Yet it is striking how little can be found in the literature that deals with the specific area of communication in the management of illness in children.

The existing literature acknowledges that pediatric communication is special in that it requires age and cognitive considerations, understanding of the complexity of the family unit, and an awareness of the fact that children are especially influenced by the environment (like the smells, sounds, and surroundings of their medical visit).

This research stems from two central disciplines: either specific sub-specialties of pediatrics such as child mental health or pediatric orthopedics, or from the specific section within the study of media and communication known as "Health Communication." Both of these promote issues such as good bedside manner and clarity of explanations, and provide practical communication tips such as "whisper," "never frown at an X-ray" or "consider using softer words."

Many pediatricians are ill-equipped to handle difficult communication situations. They don't always know how to express sympathy; they avoid or delay the most difficult conversations with children and parents, or ruin them with awkwardness or insensitivity, causing parents lasting emotional distress. For lack of a coherent semantic perspective (like the one attempted here), in the best of cases, doctors are provided with lists of "dos and don'ts." They are told they should ask what the family knows and understands, speak slowly and without using medical jargon, turn off beepers or phones, allow silence and tears, and avoid the urge to talk to overcome their own discomfort. Saying "I know how you feel" is discouraged in favor of "this must be very difficult for you."

All of this advice is what once used to be called "common sense." But, apparently, one cannot count on it being so today, based on the staggering statistics reflecting malpractice claims (especially in the United States).

One way to gauge semantic iatrogenesis is through malpractice claims. According to Levinson (1997), several studies have explored what kinds of breakdowns in communication contribute to malpractice claims. She quotes one study by Beckman and colleagues that examined malpractice depositions and identified communication problems between physicians and patients in 70% of the cases they reviewed. The communication problems they identified were of four types: deserting the patient, devaluing patients' views, delivering information poorly, and failing to understand patients' or families' perspectives.

One of the realms in which these problems in the pediatric semantic environment are most visible, is the medical interview. All practicing physicians spend a significant amount of each day talking with patients and families. In fact, the medical interview is a practicing doctor's most common procedure. According to Levinson (1997), many physicians conduct a hundred medical interviews in a week and more than 150,000 interviews during their careers. She explains further that good communication skills optimize the quality of the medical interview, enhancing patient satisfaction and improving actual health outcomes. And she emphasizes that the pediatric interview is more complicated than the traditional adult-patient medical interview since it is usually conducted with at least two people, the patient and the parent. She believes that doctors should tailor the interview to involve the child maximally (according to age or developmental stage), while attending to the needs of the parent or other family members, so that they don't leave the pediatrician's office without having shared their concerns.

All this is, of course, very good advice. But it doesn't add up to a coherent theory of pediatric communication. A wider semantic perspective is required. Just as Jacobi (the doctor credited as the founder of pediatrics) advocated a broad perspective on child health and disease prevention, and not a narrow one focused on disease, so we advocate here, on the basis of General Semantics, a view of pediatric care as an entire ecology or a semantic environment and not only as a medical specialty. This may help prevent semantic iatrogenic disease.

CHAPTER 3
The Communication Panacea:
Pediatrics and General Semantics

———■———

For each illness that doctors cure with medicine, they
provoke ten in healthy people by inoculating them with
the virus that is a thousand times more powerful than
any microbe:
the idea that one is ill.

—Marcel Proust

"THE MAP IS NOT the territory" is perhaps the most central idea of General Semantics. In *Science and Sanity*, Korzybski (1958) explains: "A map is not the territory it represents, but, if correct, it has a similar structure to the territory, which accounts for its usefulness." And he continues: "If we reflect upon our languages, we find that at best they must be considered only as maps; a word is not the object it represents" (p. 58). Or, as Hayakawa (1963) puts it, "Words, and whatever words may suggest, are not the things they stand for" (p. 22). And, in discussing this idea, Korzybski distinguishes between the structure and the content of a language:

> If words are not things, or maps are not the actual territory, then, obviously, the only possible link between the objective world and the linguistic world is found in structure and structure alone. The only usefulness of map or a language depends on the

similarity of structure between the empirical world and the map-languages. (p. 61)

Connecting General Semantics and Media Ecology, semantic and media environments, Korzybski and McLuhan, Strate (2011) discusses the relationship between the inner environment of the map, and the outer environment of the territory. And he explains that it is along this relationship that Korzybski made reference to verbal and semantic environments, and Neil Postman to media as environments. The relationship between the map and the territory is the relationship between the medium and the message, between the structure or context of the semantic environment and its content.

To understand the semantic environment of pediatrics it is important to understand both its context and its content. We turn our attention first to its context, as it is the symbolic form, the nature or the structure of a semantic environment that is most significant. As Strate (2008) puts it, "it is the materials that we work with and the methods we use to work with them, that have the most to do with the final outcome of our labors."

THE CONTEXT OF THE PEDIATRIC SEMANTIC ENVIRONMENT: PURPOSES, RELATIONSHIPS AND EMOTIONS

What makes the medical encounter successful or conducive to healing or coping is not just the language people use in it, but the relationship of what they say to the totality of the situation they are in. The totality of the semantic environment, as Postman (1976) describes it, includes people, their purposes, principles and performance (or how the purposes and principles combine). In the semantic environment of pediatrics, the people are the doctor, the parent and the child. The purposes are officially or formally, to cure and to heal although, as we shall discuss further on, there are additional, more informal purposes such as the parent needing someone to listen to them and understand them; the principles guiding the situation are the parents' responsibility to care for their children and the professional and ethical rules of medicine; and performance is the end result--the cure--and more importantly, the process that allows or does not allow for all the participants' purposes--aside from the cure--to be achieved. All of this constitutes the context of pediatrics.

In order to combine well with the principles of the situation, language should be used ecologically--inside the context in which it is used. By knowing only what a patient or her parents have said, the doctor does not know enough to judge its meaning, and it is therefore not helpful or functional. If doctors understand the context (the reality of the patient at home, the parents' relationship amongst themselves, the experiences of the child at school), they understand the specific situation and therefore the purposes of the patients and families using the language, too.

People play many different roles and they have many kinds of purposes, so they inhabit different semantic environments, each with special rules by which people are expected to conduct themselves. There's the home semantic environment, work and school, among others, and there is also the different medical environments of the hospital or the doctor's clinic, for prevention or for cures. Each of these is a social structure in which people want to do something for, with or against other people, as well as to, for, with, or against themselves.

However, sometimes in the medical encounter there are conflicting purposes. Since almost every human situation – and certainly medicine – involves at least two people, every semantic environment is generated by and organized around not one purpose but several. As Postman (1976) puts it, "semantic environments are multi-purposed" (p. 21).

Korzybski suggests that we use language the way science does. He insists that the language of science (objective, detached, unambiguous, public and tentative), is the language of sanity. But, as Postman suggests, sanity has more forms of expression than can be encompassed in one single semantic environment. "The language of prayer" he says, "is not scientific, but only in the most impoverished conception of the human enterprise can it be called insane" (p.23). And such is the case in medicine, too. On the face of it, medicine is an endeavor close to science, as it uses its principles to discover the biological sources and causes of illness as well as to develop the medications necessary to cure it. But that is not all that medicine is.

As Postman also explains, there can be no meaningful concept of either good or bad language without respect to purpose. And in multi-purposed situations such as a visit to the pediatrician, language, to be good, must also be emotional, subjective, and empathic. Patients may listen to the scientific language of the doctor and act according to her orders, but also combine prayer or find solace in narratives of, for example, love. "Good talk is talk that does what it is supposed to do in a particular situation," (p.24) and medicine is a situation that is not supposed only to physically heal an organ but to achieve the humane end of accompanying, helping to cope, etc.

The semantic environment of medicine does not entirely belong to the doctor. True, like other environments, medicine too, has a tradition in which rules are distilled from its conventions. But disagreements are to be expected, unless doctor, parent and child all reach an agreement about purposes. Differing perceptions of the purposes of the medical encounter may stem from the difference between the hypothetical or stated purposes of the profession generally, and the achieved purposes of specific patients. This gap can be the source of great distress. But the distress can be diminished if, aside from making everybody's purposes explicit, doctors understand and therefore control, tone, atmosphere, attitude, and all other the elements that define relationships and that, in turn, define the emotional context of a semantic environment.

Patients have little control over the tone--the atmosphere and attitude-- or the ambiance and texture of the semantic environment. But doctors have great control over it. Especially in the case of children, pediatricians should be aware of the level of noise, they should consider their dress and not necessarily insist on wearing their white or green robes; they should pay attention to the arrangement of the furniture, to their movements, and to the types of side activities going on such as looking at a computer instead of at the child's face when talking to them; and to talk to them, as well as to the parents, of course.

When talking to children or their adult parents or guardians, doctors should pay attention to their intonation, to their form of address, to their non-verbal gestures, groans, sighs, pauses, to their frowns while looking at an x-ray, and their "hmm" when the mother or father are talking so that it is in response to what they are saying and not a clear sign of their not listening.

In an environment with a structure such as the medical environment, sensitivity is necessary to the pecking order, or the role structure of the situation. At the doctor's the role structure is quite fixed. The doctor is the authority and the patient and her parents need her expertise. As Postman claims "role structures are exceedingly resistant to change...because they give an essential stability to the situation" (p.47). But awareness of doctors to the patient's perception of the role of the situation may create a better atmosphere. And they can challenge the structure of the relationship themselves without threatening their own authority.

Knowing how to do this is especially important today. With medical information available to all on the Internet, patients are better informed than they ever were. Some of these informed patients now request to be partners with their doctors in deciding what course of treatment should be taken. Some others are "knowledge-acquirers" for whom doctors can be providers of "internet prescriptions"-- information about trustworthy sources and internet sites to learn more about the illness diagnosed. In either case, it is clear that the Internet alters patient-physician relationships and creates a new context or structure for the semantic environment.

The context of the semantic environment is also partly comprised of the types of sentences used in it. Some sentences are prescriptive, instructing both patients and their parents what to do, thus the word "prescription." Yet others are evaluative – about things that patients do that are good or bad. The function of each of these types of sentences influences both their tone and their level of abstraction.

There's a time for specificity and a time for abstraction. As Postman so humorously puts it, "if you ask how to get to 5th avenue, you do not expect to hear that to get there will be like a journey of the soul." But some areas require semantic flexibility and the ability to combine specific and general, low and high levels of abstraction. Pediatrics is such an area. To the question "what does my child have?" a cold and specific answer such as "MS," not combined with sentences that express emotion and sympathy is inappropriate, crass, and insensible. In cases of terminal disease, the patient may need--in the absence of ends--to hear about the means; about the journey of the soul in the process of coping.

Human purposes are very complex. Concern and humanism on the part of the doctor can be combined with professionalism. It takes sensitivity and control of one's language for doctors to temper their talk. "...Communication is most sensibly viewed as a means through which desirable ends may be achieved. As an end in itself, it is disappointing, even meaningless," (Postman, 1976, p. 102) and in the semantic environment of pediatrics, potentially iatrogenic.

THE CONTENT OF THE PEDIATRIC SEMANTIC ENVIRONMENT: DEFINITIONS AND DIAGNOSES, METAPHORS AND CAUSES

In the chapter titled "The Indians have no word for it" in his book *People in Quandaries*, Wendell Johnson (1946) tells of a man who pointed out that he seldom if ever stuttered when alone but only when speaking to other people, so that whatever the causes of his disorder, they must lie in those other people quite as much as in himself. According to Johnson, the man was pointing a finger in the direction of a semantic environment – "the environment of attitudes and evaluations, opinions and beliefs-as a source of his difficulties." (pp. 440-441) In other words, the aspects of the environment most important in relation to stuttering are semantic or evaluational.

To illustrate this point, Johnson talks about the fact that there are no stutterers among what we call Native Americans and he refers to as Indians. And he explains that this is apparently because of the semantic environment among them. He found in his study that their standards of child care and training were more lax in comparison with White Americans'. And in respect to speech in particular, he says that every Indian child was regarded as a satisfactory or normal speaker, regardless of the manner in which the child spoke. Speech defects were simply not recognized. The Native American children were not criticized or evaluated on the basis of their speech, no comments were made about it, and no issue was made of it. In their semantic environments there appeared to be no speech anxieties or tensions for the Indian children to interiorize, to adopt as their own.

Thus, Johnson points out, there is no word for stuttering in Native Americans' languages.

As opposed to this situation among Native Americans, it was discovered that most of the White children investigated had begun to stutter at or before the age of three years and two months and all them had talked without stuttering for from six months to several years before the onset of stuttering. And this, he explains, points directly to the semantic environment as the source of the problem. Practically every case of stuttering was originally diagnosed as such by a layperson--usually the child's parents. What they had diagnosed as stuttering was not different from the repetitions characteristic of the normal speech of young children. These repetitions seem to occur under the regular conditions in the speaking experience of young children, such as when the child lacks sufficient knowledge of the subject she is talking about, when the listener does not respond readily to what the child says, when her vocabulary does not contain yet the necessary words, or when the child is talking in the face of competition from siblings, for example. And they are not accompanied by any apparent anxiety on the part of the child.

In other words, the so-called stuttering children were found to have been normal when someone, usually the parents, first regarded them as stutterers. And they had all talked for considerable periods without being regarded as having a problem before they had come to be diagnosed as stutterers. Stuttering as a clinical problem or as a disorder was found to occur not before being diagnosed, but after. Johnson calls this kind of problem "diagnosogenic" – when the diagnosis causes the disorder. And it is one kind among many of what we call here "semantic iatrogenesis."

The disorder is a vicious spiral and an example of the iatrogenic disease commonly known as a self-fulfilling prophecy. It develops because the valuations made by the parents by diagnosing their child's speech as "stuttering" or as "defective" or "abnormal," are a very important part of the child's semantic environment. The child interiorizes this aspect of his semantic environment, and comes to evaluate his speech as "defective," himself. His speech is, in turn, made more hesitant and cautious. This makes the parents even more anxious which leads them to urge the child to "go slowly," to "stop and start over," or to "make up his mind." The more fearful and disheartened the child becomes and the more hesitantly he speaks, the more worried the parents and teachers become, and the more insistently they appeal to the child to "talk better," with the result that the child's own evaluation becomes still more disturbed, and his speech becomes more and more disordered.

General Semantics doesn't only point out what the sources of our problems are. It is both a theoretical and a practical system the proponents of which hold that its adoption can reliably alter human behavior. And so, there are actions that can be taken to better the situation. And these actions mostly concern the semantic environment. As Johnson (1946) explains, in the case of stuttering, there needs to be a change in the attitudes and policies of the parents and teachers concerning the child as a person and as a speaker. A semantic environment needs to be created for the child, in which there is a minimum of anxiety, tension and disapproval for him to interiorize; an environment that permits him to speak spontaneously, with pleasure, and with confidence. In a way, the solution is found in the inversion of the spiral: As the child senses that his speech is approved, his reluctance to speak and his exaggerated hesitancy and caution in speaking decrease. And the result is free and spontaneous speech, and a more affectionate and friendly relationship between the parents and their child. It is a matter of changing the child's speech responses by changing the relevant features of the conditions under which they occur or, as Johnson puts it:

> Anything that can be done to change the semantic environment, to modify attitudes and policies in the home, school, neighborhood or community, or to educate "public opinion" in the larger sense, helps to promote favorable changes in the individual's own evaluative behavior. (p. 454)

And this seems to us exactly what is necessary in today's pediatric semantic environment. Like "stuttering" in the 1940's when Johnson was writing about it, there are other diagnoses--of a semantic iatrogenic nature-- that plague pediatrics today.

ADHD is one of the most illustrative examples of a pediatric ailment at least partly created by diagnostic labels requiring a change in the semantic environment--of school, home, the pediatrician's office and, really, culture itself.

As in the case of stuttering, ADHD is very often diagnosed by laypersons--parents and teachers--and not by experts. And this leads to the kind of spiral described by Johnson (1946). Teachers diagnose children as having ADHD, they speak to parent who, out of concern, request medications from pediatricians, and pediatricians are sometimes too quick to comply. In turn, parents are relieved of the guilt that the child's difficulties may be due to their inadequate parenting skills, and this masks the real family entanglements that might be contributing to the over-stimulating environment that is the reason for the child's behavior.

In an opinion piece published in New York Times Sunday Review on January 28, 2012 under the title *Ritalin Gone Wrong*, psychiatrist Alan Sroufe points out that at the time of his writing, three million children in the United States were taking drugs for problems in focusing. And that toward the end of the previous year, many of their parents were deeply alarmed because there was a shortage of drugs like Ritalin and Adderall that they considered absolutely essential to their children's functioning. While acknowledging that some kids could benefit from short-term drug treatment, large-scale, long-term treatment for millions of children is not the answer. He believes that the large-scale medication of children feeds into a societal view that all of life's problems can be solved with a pill and gives millions of children the impression that there is something inherently defective in them. And alluding to the semantic environment created by this approach, he adds:

> The illusion that children's behavior problems can be cured with drugs prevents us as a society from seeking the more complex solutions that will be necessary. Drugs get everyone--politicians, scientists, teachers and parents--off the hook. Everyone except the children, that is.

Some doctors have gone as far as suggesting that to begin to alleviate the problem we need to do away with the diagnosis of ADHD. Dr. Steve Balt is one such doctor. In a blog he published on February 8th 2012 in *KevinMD.com*--a prominent social media platform on health and medicine--he explains that if we eliminate the diagnosis of ADHD, we can still evaluate children with attention or concentration problems, or hyperactivity, and we can still use stimulant medications to provide relief. Doctors do this all the time, he says. But the present situation is such that, while exceptions exist, often the diagnosis of ADHD and the prescription of a drug, that in many cases works surprisingly well, is the end of the story. Without the label or the formal diagnosis, doctors may avoid the spiral (or self-fulfilling prophecy) of a child being diagnosed, taking medication, doing better with peers or in school, parents being satisfied, and everyone forgetting about what caused the symptoms in the first place, and take care of those underlying causes.

The underlying cause may be a chaotic home environment, a history of neglect, substance abuse, a parenting style not fit for the child's social make-up. And yes, for a few it may stem from a biological abnormality. And each should be approached and treated differently. Otherwise, as Dr. Allen Francis puts it (in a *Huffington Post* piece on April 1st, 2014), we are turning childhood itself into an illness: "Our kids are no sicker now than they have always been, he says. It's just that they are too often mislabeled for behaviors that used to be considered part of normal variation." And of the latest label or diagnosis (or the new ADHD)--"sluggish cognitive tempo"-- he says (in a *KevinMD.com* piece on April 12th, 2014):

> ...SCT is a remarkably silly name for an even sillier proposal. Its main characteristics are vaguely described but include some combination daydreaming, lethargy and slow mental processing. Its proponents estimate that SCT afflicts approximately two million children. Not surprisingly, Eli Lilly is already on the case.

And he adds: "...Possibly the very dumbest and most dangerous diagnostic idea I have ever encountered."

Diagnoses of stuttering, ADHD, sluggish cognitive tempo and others in both adults and children are definitions that are coined by doctors and researchers, gain acceptance, become cultural paradigms and alter the semantic environment. And they are one of General Semantics' most central terms.

"What meanings we give to the world, what sense we make of things" Postman (1976) says, "derive from our power to name, to create vocabularies." And he adds that in discussing what words we shall use in describing an event, we are not engaging in "mere semantics." We are engaged in trying to control the perceptions and responses of others (as well as ourselves) to the character of the event itself. This is the source of the power of the medical establishment, of systems of health, of doctors generally, and pediatricians specifically. It is the power to name that gives them their status. And when that power is abused, they commit what Postman calls "Definition Tyranny."

In spite of the commonplace, one cannot tell anything "like it is." Things aren't anything until someone names them. The way in which they are named reveals not the way they are but how the namer wishes to see them or how she is capable of seeing them. How something has been named becomes the reality not only for the namer, but also of all who accept the name. Doctors and researchers created a category, compiled under it a myriad of processes and conditions, and labeled it stuttering or ADHD, and millions of people around the world found themselves in a new reality-- a new semantic environment.

The new reality does not need to be everyone's reality. Postman encourages us to ask ourselves what the nature of the reality that the namer's words create is, what response do the words require of us, and does our response serve our purposes or at least purposes with which we agree.

An illustration of the rejection of the reality created by the medical establishment's naming or definitions can be found in a piece by Richard Saul in *The New Republic* on February 14th, 2014 titled *ADHD Does Not Exist* (also the title of his book). He says:

> You might be saying to yourself, okay, ADHD is
> probably over-diagnosed. And yes, some people who
> are on a stimulant probably shouldn't be, like the

college student struggling to focus on a boring lecture or the kid who's fidgeting a bit too much for his teacher's liking. But how can it be that among the millions of people diagnosed—over 4 percent of adults and 11 percent of children in the U.S.—not one of them actually has ADHD? Because we've all encountered someone with severe attention or hyperactivity issues—the boy who is always daydreaming, the girl who gets out of her seat to run around the room while her classmates sit calmly, the woman who consistently asks questions that have just been answered. Surely at least some of these people have ADHD! Actually, not one of them does. Let me be clear: In my view, not a single individual— not even the person who finds it close to impossible to pay attention or sit still—is afflicted by the disorder called ADHD as we define it today.

You may have noticed that Saul points to the definition of ADHD as the basis for his statement that "it" does not exist. He explains that he finds the way we define this "illness" striking, because, unlike other illnesses, it is an illness defined by its symptoms, rather than its cause.

If we were to define a heart attack by chest pain, then the appropriate cure would be painkillers, rather than the revival and repair of the heart...Nasal congestion can be a symptom of a cold, allergy, or many other conditions, but a runny nose is not a diagnosis. In the same way, the symptom complex associated with the ADHD diagnosis is related to more than twenty medical diagnoses (from those as mild as poor eyesight, sleep deprivation, and even boredom in the classroom, to more severe conditions like depression and bipolar disorder), that, when treated effectively, can result in the disappearance of the attention-deficit and hyperactivity symptoms.

The question is, of course, whose interest it is in to use the label of ADHD and provide treatment for it or its symptoms and not their causes. Who is in charge – if we allow it – of the definition of reality in the pediatric semantic environment?

According to Saul, the symptoms of distractibility and impulsivity are all too real, but we're using an outdated, invalid definition of ADHD, that has been kept in place for decades by physicians and other practitioners, pharmaceutical companies, the media, and even patients themselves--the millions of falsely diagnosed patients for whom the reality includes also delayed or denied treatment, spiraling health-care costs, significant health risks and frustration.

On the basis of the same logic as Johnson's, what Saul is advocating is paying attention to what the definition of ADHD has done to the semantic environment, and acting accordingly: To change the attitudes and policies of parents and teachers concerning the child; to create a semantic environment for the child at school and at home that permits her to concentrate; to change the relevant features of the conditions under which boredom and restlessness occur.

What both Johnson and Saul are aware of--as is clear from even the titles of their works (*The Indians Have No Word For It* and *ADHD Does Not Exist*)--is that "the word is not the thing," which cannot be said of some of the doctors and other health professionals whose responses to the phrase "ADHD does not exist" were signal responses – automatic and emotional – confusing the map with the territory.

As we have shown to this point, the language of each social structure expresses human purpose through its tone, its vocabulary, and its levels of abstraction. But another central aspect of the content of a semantic environment is its metaphors.

Metaphors impose a precise kind of imagery or point of view on a situation and when there is no awareness to them people's perceptions get locked into a particular way of construing what is happening. The field of medicine, as Postman (1976) explains:

> ...relies to a considerable extent on the idea that disease is an alien force that "attacks" or "invades" human beings. Some diseases are best described this way, but there are many others which require a different metaphor altogether...Do we really "catch" a cold or do we "manufacture" it? Do we "contract" TB or "concoct" it? In the instance of ulcers, most of us are prepared to believe that we do not "catch" it; we "produce" it. But what of arthritis, cancer, rheumatism? The search for cures will depend, to a large extent, on our finding new and illuminating metaphors. (p. 66)

The metaphorical biases of semantic environments are not always destructive, but they are apt to be hard to see and require close scrutiny to avoid committing ourselves to a point of view of which we are not always aware. When we internalize the metaphors conventionally used to describe our children's health or illnesses, we are unable to imagine different metaphors being applied. Our perceptions are completely controlled by someone else's metaphors. We are then at the mercy of our doctors' or even our cultures' point of view. But if we are able of conceiving alternative metaphors, the better we get at controlling our responses to the situation.

One of the classic examples of metaphors controlling people's responses to illness is found in Sontag's book on the metaphors used to talk and think about tuberculosis and cancer. Sontag (1988) traced the development of the social narrative of tuberculosis in the 19th century and paralleled it with a 20th century narrative of cancer. Both diseases have a clear medical origin and, as Sontag points out, share metaphoric meanings that make attributions about their sufferers that may lead to additional problems. Tuberculosis was initially viewed as a disease of the artist--primarily afflicting a person of sensitive and sad temperament--and later as a product of urban moral decay and sexual excess. Cancer is still sometimes viewed as a disease of suppressed or concealed emotions that must be "fought," "defeated," and removed. Both social narratives affected the experiences of those unfortunate enough to have contracted these diseases and sometimes even led to treatment regimens not altogether helpful to the healing process. Sontag expanded her thesis in a later book (1989) to include AIDS in the discussion.

The martial metaphors that Sontag discusses have become so ingrained in our public discourse, that it has become close to impossible not to use them. From the news, to advertising to our everyday talk, it is hard to find utterances about disease and public health that manage to avoid words like "campaign," "target," weapon," "battle," "fight," or "crusade."

This is significant because, as JoAnne Brown (as quoted by Dale Keiger, 1998) explains, if enough people think of a public health effort as a war on disease, it is then easier to enact policies that curtail civil liberties, for example. A war is, after all, a crisis and, as such, it sometimes calls for extraordinary measures. The use of the language of war gives priority to the crisis, and trivializes other concerns. Brown is convinced that public health policies that were meant to separate carriers of tuberculosis from the general public, eventually helped legitimize racist measures like the statutory segregation of drinking fountains.

The detection of the metaphors underlying public and professional discourse on pediatrics is very important. Pediatricians often use the phrase, "children are not just small adults." This, as Gillis and Loughlan (2007) assert, may be a useful idea for the calculation of drug doses and the assessment of physiological parameters. But the definition of child medicine in such negative and exclusionary terms carries with it some inherent dangers and misconceptions. And they explain that both children and adults belong to the human race; that progress in medicine can usually be applied to and be of benefit to all; that the transition from childhood to adulthood should be one of continuity rather than migration; and that by emphasizing that children are not small adults, doctors unconsciously negate all that may be gained through a vision which considers human beings throughout their lives.

The authors suggest that one way to find alternative metaphors is to look back at earlier stages of pediatrics to see how early practitioners tried to impart what they took as the unique qualities of their specialty. Then, at the end of the 19th century and the beginning of the 20th, two main metaphors were employed: the pediatrician as veterinary or the pediatrician as explorer, both based on the lack of ability to obtain direct patient history, because of infants' incapacity to describe their own feelings.

The authors quote a British doctor, Sir James Goodhart, who practiced at Evelina Hospital for Children in London from 1875 to 1889, and wrote a book in 1885 where he concluded:

> Yet there is not so very much difference between the student who has to investigate the diseases of children, and one who has to deal with those of the

lower animals. In both cases the diagnosis will chiefly rest upon the doctor's personal observation and examination; in both it is intelligible speech that is wanting.

Gillis and Loughlan (2007) explain further that the veterinary analogy reinforced the need for doctors to improve their capabilities in the direct clinical assessment of child patients. And they add that the veterinary analogy also fit the observations at the time about the animal characteristics of young children, which it was felt "recapitulated" the evolution of the species. Ernst Haeckel's recapitulation theory claimed that the development of each individual repeats the stages of development of the species. Many authors applied the theory to child development, revealing past atavisms in a baby's reflexes and child behavior. Thus baby and infant development was easily equated with animal development.

The explorer metaphor was another way of handling the absence of a first person patient history, and the physical signs were given the status of a language. The language metaphor was adopted in 1845 by the French pediatrician, Eugene Bouchut, and he is quoted as saying that the physician who examines a child cannot derive anything from the insufficient language of the child and so he must have recourse to the language given to the child by God, or what philosophers call natural language--the language of signs. And Thomas Rotch, the doctor that held the first Chair in pediatrics at Harvard, took the explorer metaphor one step further, beyond language, to an alien culture. In his 1891 presidential address to the American Pediatric Society he described the experience of child medicine for his colleagues:

"We have entered upon the especial investigation of and research in this branch of anthropology with the keen interests of explorers in an almost unknown country."

The explorer and the veterinary metaphors tried to make sense of the absence of speech and the resulting reliance on physical signs. And Gillis and Loughlan believe there are resonances of these metaphors in pediatric practice to this day. They believe that recognition of the metaphors may help doctors make sense of their responses to children and their parents.

Like all metaphors, these historical metaphors are not neutral, and they have hidden meanings and implications, thus they shape how pediatricians conceive the essence of their practice.

Metaphors have aided physicians greatly in their understanding of what the healthy body is and how it survives and protects itself. It was probably hard to make sense of the heart before we knew what a pump was; and automatic gun turrets helped to explain the finesse of voluntary muscular movement. These are, on the face of it, technical metaphors. But like metaphors, if extended, they carry with them entire narratives. As Gillis and Loughlan (2007) put it:

> The veterinary metaphor connotes the importance of the objective abilities of the physician, with the child to be understood from an observational, passive and non-empathetic distance. The explorer metaphor is adventurous and exciting, recognises that these are human beings and suggests a more engaged approach requiring active learning of a culture and language. (p. 947)

In other words, veterinary medicine and explorations are not only metaphors, they are entire narratives.

When medicine becomes important as it is today, people are from birth to death involved in medical rituals and the rituals have one social purpose: generating narratives or myths, such as the narrative based on the metaphor of "pain-killing." But as Illich (1976) explains, painkilling hasn't always been the leading narrative. The pupils of Hippocrates distinguished many kinds of disharmony, each of which caused its own kind of pain. And so, pain became a useful tool for diagnosis. It revealed to the physician which harmony the patient had to recover. Pain could disappear in the process of healing, but this was not the primary goal of the doctor's treatment. Pain was the soul's experience of evolution. The human body was part of an irreparably impaired universe, and the soul postulated by Aristotle was coextensive with his body. In this narrative, there was no need to distinguish between the sense and the experience of pain. All words that indicated bodily pain were equally applicable to the suffering of the soul.

Nowadays, the narrative is a very different one and its metaphors have very different consequences. In pediatrics, as Illich (1976) puts it:

> The sickness that society produces is baptized by the doctor with names that bureaucrats cherish. "Learning disability," "hyperkinesis," or "minimal brain dysfunction" explains to parents why their children do not learn, serving as an alibi for school's intolerance or incompetence. (p. 61)

The concept of narrative has played a central role in various fields during the past two decades or so. Clandinin and Caine (2008) for example, explain that narrative inquiry is first and foremost a way of understanding experience. But it is also a research methodology. In other words, it is both a view of people's experiences and a methodology for inquiring into experience, through narrative, and thus allows for the intimate study of individuals' experiences over time and in context. Beginning with a narrative view of experience, researchers attend to place, temporality, and sociality, allowing for inquiry into both researchers' and participants' storied life experiences. Within this space, each story told and lived is situated and understood within larger cultural, social, and institutional narratives. Narrative inquiry is marked by its emphasis on relational engagement between researcher and research participants, and as it is already clear here, in the context of medicine, between doctor and patient.

Narrative inquiry, across various disciplines and multiple professional fields, aims at understanding and making meaning of experience through conversations, dialogue, and participation in the ongoing lives of the participants. Each discipline and field of study brings slightly different ways of understanding and different contexts--or semantic environments--to the narrative study of experience.

Pollio et al. (2006) explain that narrative analysis begins with the assumption that one way to learn something about a person, group, or culture is to consider the stories they tell. It addresses how stories guide personal and social meanings and views human life as a text that can be analyzed much as literary critics analyze their texts.

The story, narrative or text provides a reconfigured version of human experience using structures available in language. The narrative is defined by its temporal structure and depends on shared cultural understandings of order and causality. Although our immediate experience of the world may not necessarily unfold as a narrative, when we reflect on it and tell it to others, it usually does assume this form.

Narrative development takes place on two levels. The first level takes place when personal experience is reconstructed emphasizing certain aspects of our world and allowing others to become context. Language provides words that direct us to some things and allow us to ignore others. We identify and isolate aspects of our experience and begin to represent it as a cluster of observations to which words can be applied. And at the second level, a story formulated as experience is shaped into an account that can be told to someone else within a specific social and historical context.

Narrative Inquiry has by now become an accepted method in many cultures and diverse academic traditions, including psychology, linguistics, education, sociology, anthropology, journalism, and political science, and, of course, medicine.

We all have a story that we tell ourselves about our healthy lives. But illness requires us to re-organize our story and therefore narratives of illness are a good way of understanding how people--as individuals and as part of a culture--deal with chronic conditions.

Charmaz (2000) also claims that experiencing chronic illness means much more than feeling physical distress, acknowledging symptoms, and needing care. It includes metaphor and meaning, moral judgments and ethical dilemmas, identity questions and reconstruction of self, daily struggles and persistent troubles. Experiencing serious illness challenges prior meanings, ways of living that have been taken for granted, and ways of knowing the self. For the ill person life is suddenly uncertain. The self becomes vulnerable, and its vulnerability derives, in part, from potential disapproval and devaluation. Chronically ill people lose their previously taken-for-granted continuity of life. And they need empowering metaphors and narratives.

Conflict between practitioners and patients can arise from unstated assumptions such as guiding metaphors. Patients have their own metaphors, values, and sentiments. Their stories mediate between their bodies and emotions because their stories make sense of their altered lives and limited bodies. They tell of change and transition, of beginnings and endings throughout adult life. Yet stories alone do not cover the experience. Not everyone can find words to express inchoate feelings. It is the doctor's job--through interviews and conversations--to find, with the patient, useful and healing metaphors and illness narratives.

Narrative strategies and poetic conventions such as voice, genre, master metaphors, and rhetorical strategies need to be taken into account, as they are essential to the way in which illness narratives are constructed. Illness narratives do not simply recount a series of disconnected events; they tell a story that is typically, a moral one. Illness is located within the autobiography of the person in question. It often contains implicit or explicit ideologies and morals that may be at odds with rationalized biomedical conventions. This is what we previously called the differing perceptions of the purposes of the medical encounter; the difference between the hypothetical or stated purposes of the profession generally, and the achieved purposes of specific patients.

And so, this approach requires a developed narrative or metaphorical sensitivity as well as personal empathy from doctors. They need to be able to hear the story that is being told and to trace the ways in which widely shared cultural conventions are taken up as the embodied metaphors of some person's life or illness.

At the same time, clinicians should realize that their own stories about illness and healing--the stories that they tell themselves, each other, and patients or their families--are also based on specific metaphors. The idea that patients should always be hopeful, that physicians should always be heroic, or conversely that "realism" requires a matter-of-fact stoicism on the part of the families of the terminally ill, are all narrative strategies that have bearing on the ways in which care is organized, resources distributed, and meanings either allowed or disallowed from the clinical encounter.

In short, as Delvecchio Good and Good (2000) succinctly put it, clinical narratives--stories of therapeutic activities created by physicians for and with patients over time--lie at the heart of doctor-patient communication. Through clinical narrative, physicians create and shape patient experience over time. And they add:

> Physicians in conversation with patients, "emplot" disease and its treatment, constructing meaningful stories, linking the past and the present to potential futures, and plotting courses of action. (p. 246)

In other words, what physicians do is time-bind. Time-binding, a key term in General Semantics, refers to what characterizes us as humans, as the only species with the unique capacity for language and symbolic communication. As time-binders, doctors can help patients maintain a sense of continuity and of permanence. As Lee (1994) puts it:

> To see the uniqueness of man's time-binding capacity is to begin to realize the significance of language. If we discover the creative uses of words, we may begin to know what it is to function humanly. (p. 5)

Time-binding and functioning humanly is what guided one of the authors of this book throughout his pediatric career. A few of the narratives he encountered along the way are told in the next chapter, with an emphasis on the semantic environments that characterized them, their context and content.

PART II

CHAPTER 4
Eight Stories: Conquering Semantic Iatrogenesis

———————

It is more important to know what sort of person has a
disease than to know what sort of disease a person has.
— Hippocrates

I N *THE HEALER'S ART*, CASSELL (1985) distinguishes between "healing" and "curing" and between two distinct aspects of sickness: the illness and the disease that caused it. He explains that if one doesn't distinguish between illness and disease, making a patient with pneumonia better, means killing the bacteria, and bringing down his fever. But there are other aspects of the illness that cannot be ignored: the patient may be frightened about what is happening in his body; he may feel cut off from his family and his friends; and he may find himself painfully dependent on other people. And handling those aspects of the patient's pneumonia is also part of the doctor's job. He says further that thanks to technology, doctors have become more effective in curing disease than at any other time in history. But this, as we mentioned in our introduction, has contributed to the weakening of healing as part of the definition of the doctor's job.

In a later book, Cassell (1997) adds another concept--"doctoring"—to the concepts of "curing" and "healing." And he explains that doctoring includes the "being" of the physician, not just the "doing." Physicians are not merely bearers of knowledge and skills, but are themselves the instruments of care. As such, they must understand how language works and how it influences the nature of relationships, as these

...will endure within physicians who practice long after the knowledge of medical science learned in medical school has become obsolete... The relief of suffering stands alongside the preservation of life. (pp. 7-8)

In yet another book--*Talking with Patients*--Cassell (1985) displays an awareness of the non-Aristotelian logic of General Semantics. He speaks, for example, of science having been successful because of the ability of scientists to study in controlled isolation, simple, linear, cause-and effect parts of more complex wholes. This, he explains, produces "dyadic" statements such as "If A, then B," or the "All or None" rule of nerve conduction. And he adds that explanatory principles are easily constructed when phenomena can be characterized in terms of dyads, or sets of dyads. Language, however, is irreducibly triadic. Words do not merely stand for things, they represent not only something "out there" but the person using them as well...Words always stand for something to someone. The irreducible triangle consists of a word, the thing it stands for, and the person for whom it has that meaning. And this, he believes, provides opportunities for clinicians, because human illness is, in fact, triadic in the same manner as language.

Moreover, Cassell seems aware of the General Semantics concepts of "dating" and "indexing," or the ideas that no two people afflicted with supposedly the same disease are ill in the same way, and that even within one patient, no two occurrences of the illness are the same. When isolated and confined to their afflicted cells, organs or enzyme systems, he says, may be quite constant in the manner in which they express themselves, and we have instruments to measure their activity. However, each illness caused by a given disease is unique, and differs from every other illness episode because of the person in whom it occurs. And even when a disease recurs in the same individual, the illness is changed by the fact that it is a recurrence; it now carries the associations and the history of the previous episode.

> Though it is obvious that genetic makeup or changes in immune response can alter the reaction to disease, as can diet, personal habits, and level of physical conditioning, the presentation, course, and outcome of a disease can also be affected by whether the patient likes or fears physicians, "believes" in medication or abuses drugs, is brave or cowardly, self-destructive or vain, has unconscious conflicts into which the illness does or does not fit, and so on. These features are part of the illness, for illness is not only a physical event but a "meaning event" as well. (Cassell, 1985, p. 6)

In a way, Cassell foresees the current revolution of Personalized Genetic Medicine, that, based on breakthroughs in our understanding of an individual's unique molecular characteristics, are making it possible to customize healthcare and personalize the diagnosis and treatment of disease at the individual patient level. But his prophecy is unique in that he emphasizes the psychological elements that influence how each person experiences a disease in his call for the personalization of medicine. No technological development can bring about the possibility of customized treatment in this sense. But a semantic awareness can, and this is the focus of the following stories or narratives.

Dr. Isaac Berger (the M.D. among the authors) always saw himself as a professional not only in the realm of curing, but also of healing and doctoring. As such, he practiced what may be called

"Personalized Semantic Medicine." In the footsteps of the long line of doctors (Cassell, 1985, 1997; Groopman, 2008; Hilfiker, 1985; among others) who, in the past three decades or so, have presented stories of disease and of illness, of curing and healing, and especially inspired by pediatrician and poet William Carlos Williams's (1984) *The Doctor Stories*, we turn now to tell eight of the stories of children encountered by Isaac over his career.

Isaac told the stories to Eva (the Ph.D. among us), and in the process, we both had an opportunity to reflect on them. This reflection, lead to our decision to formulate the stories together, referring to the doctor in the third person rather than in the form of either a first-hand rendition or an interview, for clarity's sake.

We tell the stories through the lens of General Semantics as, as Postman (1976) explains, an awareness of its central concepts (or what he calls a meta-semantic strategy), allows us to put ourselves, psychologically, outside the context of the semantic environment so that we may see its entirety, or at least see it from multiple perspectives. This is not only done in hindsight, as throughout his career, Isaac insisted on moving from being a participant to being a participant-observer. In recounting the stories of a few of his patients here, we bring to the surface his assumptions, his grammatical biases, and the metaphorical structure of his doctoring, in hope that this will encourage other doctors to reflect on the character of their semantic environments, without fear of this awareness jeopardizing the stability and continuity of their work. To be aware of what's going on in the hospital or at the clinic does not imply that one will refuse to do and say what one is supposed to, on the contrary. As Postman puts it:

> The greater one's awareness of the purposes and
> structures of our semantic environments, the greater

is one's sensitivity to the precariousness of all social order...of all communication. To discover that what keeps us together is nothing more substantial than a curious set of symbols and a delicate system of rules is more likely to lead one to humility...than to...rebelliousness. (p. 239)

The meta-semantic view advanced here, has the potential of freeing doctors from both ritualistic compliance and reflexive rejection. Once free, they may reenter the situation (or refuse to reenter it) from an entirely different point of view and with a heightened degree of control. We achieve capabilities of critical, self-conscious, rational, delayed and provisional responses. And this leads to empathy, responsibility and civility – all that is worth preserving in the semantic environment of pediatrics.

CARPE DIEM: AMI'S METAPHOR

The role of metaphor in human thought and, therefore, in our conceptions and explanation of the world and our experience, has been studied extensively in fields such as linguistics and philosophy. Lakoff and Johnson (1980) talk about the pervasiveness of metaphors in thought as well as in action and explain that they are a characteristic of our everyday functioning. They don't define metaphor as "mere" ornament of speech and style, and rather see it as the verbal aspect of a deeper process of cognition. Our thoughts and our actions, they believe, are fundamentally metaphorical in nature.

In this sense, simple verbs such as "to be" or "to do" are powerful metaphors which express some of our most fundamental conceptions of the way things are. As Postman (1976) explains, we believe that there are things that people "have" and others that people "do," and others still that people "are." Just as every legal system and every moral code is based on a set of assumptions about what people "are," "have," or "do," and any significant changes in law or morality are preceded by a reordering of how such metaphors are employed, so doctors who "play" with these verbs, and channel the dialogue in the direction of one or the other of these metaphors, can make great changes in how illness is conceptualized by parents and children. Control over these metaphors means control over the situation. Aware of this and of the transactional nature of our existence, Isaac himself talks about the time when he "made" his heart attack.

The story of Ami is a story of the triumph of the metaphor of "having sickness" over the metaphor of "being sick." Ami understood, and made it clear to his mother and to Isaac, that as opposed to "smart," for example, which he felt was something he "was," illness was something he "had." The spinal muscular atrophy is what killed him in the end, alright, but it was not who he was. It was something he had, along with many other things. Who he was, was the healthiest person all the people who knew him, including his doctor, ever knew.

Ami's story is an especially illuminating example of the coping power of metaphors, as the relationship between doctor, patient and parent lasted 32 years, and bore, throughout those years, metaphors that can be said to have been, at least partly, responsible for the chronically ill patient's unusually long life and, more importantly, the quality of his life in his own eyes.

Isaac first met Ami at the age of ten. He was born with spinal muscular atrophy and was confined to a wheelchair since the age of four. Isaac became his pediatrician and followed him very closely until Ami's demise at the age of 41.

Because of his physical impairment and his mother's inability to move him around, he became one of the few patients in Isaac's practice for whom he made house-calls when these were already a thing of the past in most places. The combination of the long-term relationship and the house calls, helped avoid some of the metaphors that are typical of the semantic environment of the doctor's clinic.

"Who can enter a doctor's office or a hospital," says Postman (1976)

> ...and construe his or her role in the situation as that of a "costumer"? Many people I know are apt to think of themselves, when sitting in a doctor's office, as a student who has been called upon to explain some difficulty to the principal. Such "patient-students" are reluctant to take too much of the "doctor-principal's" time, they do not address him by his first name, they do not ask questions, they are eager to do exactly as they are told, and if the doctor tells them that he can see nothing wrong with the ear of which they have complained, they are apologetic about having mentioned it in the first place. (p.127)

The familiar environment of home, in the days when house-calls were the rule, inherently avoided these kinds of metaphors, as doctors could not sustain such a metaphor outside their offices. But as house-calls are the exception to the rule these days, doctors should keep this matter in mind and not generate such metaphors. This can be avoided, for example, by designing the office or the clinic in a way that dissipates any sense of mystery, anxiety and guilt that places such as a school principal's office invariably do, or by a simple gesture such as apologizing when summoning a patient late.

Every semantic environment is projected as being something other than it is. And the way we construe a situation, the metaphor we use to think about it, determines how we conduct ourselves. So it is important for doctors to set a good leading metaphor. Pediatricians understand this better than any other kind of doctors. Many of them have drawings on their clinics' walls, they avoid white or green robes, they have little toys and candy to give out, and when they are semantically savvy, the language to go with the metaphor of their office or clinic as kindergarten or playground.

Isaac estimates that about 50% of his visits (which were innumerable) were initiated by Ami or his mother simply wanting to talk, needing psychological support and not medical care in its narrow sense. Isaac spoke to Ami and tried to answer his every question. He never lied. He told him of his prospects and explained each element of his condition, but always tried to not let his own personal and professional narratives, values and metaphors override Ami's. Through their conversations, Isaac tried to help Ami use his own metaphors and create his own empowering illness narrative. And indeed, he did.

While living in the United States for a while, Ami's mother was told by a doctor that Ami wouldn't survive beyond the age of six. He lived to the age of 41, and lived a rich and fulfilling life. With his bodily motion limited to a single finger on his left hand, Ami was a talented 3-D animator. He fell in love with his caretaker, was always surrounded by friends, went out to drink with them (sipping from a straw), participated in their conversation using a Madonna style microphone to amplify his voice and amusing them with his great sense of humor, and dreamed of riding a Harley Davidson.

Isaac tried to maintain the open-ended narrative approach to the interpersonal context and effects of Ami's illness. He tried to always stay in tune with whatever Ami--the maker and teller of the narrative--considered to be at stake. He tried to listen carefully to his hopes, fears and personal history, and accommodate them. But this lead to one of the only conflicts Isaac encountered-- not with Ami, but with his mother.

After examining Ami and talking to him, Isaac was routinely invited by Ami's mother to join her in the kitchen for a cup of coffee and for what Isaac eventually realized to be the weaving of Ami's story through the years in her mind. But this time, she thought Isaac's acceptance of Ami's story had gone too far.

At the age of about 30 and weighing 39 pounds, Ami decided to take a trip to the United States in search of the neurologist who told his mother when he was three that Ami would die before he reached six years of age. His mother objected to this and argued that Ami was not strong enough to survive the trip. But Ami insisted. So making sure that all the necessary measures were taken by his friends and that they had a plan what to do in case of an emergency, Isaac supported Ami's plans and provided instructions.

When two or more people within a semantic environment construct different and incompatible metaphors of the situation, conflict ensues. This is what happened at first. But Isaac became the translator, mediator or elucidator, making explicit in their conversations Ami's underlying metaphors and narrative for life. Ami, his mother and Isaac ended up functioning within the same metaphorical framework. So much so, that the mother joined Ami for part of the journey.

Ami took the trip with his friends. They rented a van, returned to Ami's birthplace in Texas for a reunion with his brother, and a motorcycle club fulfilled his dream and gave him a chance to ride in the sidecar of a Harley. The trip was documented by one his friends-- an Israeli film director--and Ami was not only the protagonist but also the animator of the film, literally constructing his own reality according to his own imagery.

Doctors need to figure out what their own metaphors are of themselves, their profession and their semantic environments, and not only facilitate or negotiate their patients' metaphors. Postman (1976) says:

> The doctor who thinks of his profession as a priestly craft will naturally think his "parishioners" arrogant if they ask too many questions or seek to penetrate the mysteries of his ministrations. The patient who thinks of himself as a "customer" will naturally think of the doctor as an arrogant businessman who has insufficient respect for those on whom his income is dependent. Both seek a good relationship, but they will not achieve it. (p.130)

The metaphors guiding our behavior compose our "life scripts." If, for example, doctors think of life as a struggle or a battle, their behavior in the semantic environments of their practice will be an adversary one. If, instead of forcing patients to accept their metaphorical construction doctors negotiate patients' and parents' metaphors, uncovering them by attending to language and noticing patterns of speech, there are better chances of having everyone in the situation reconstruct it along the lines of what is in the patient's best interest.

A certain measure of compliance is required to make a metaphor work. As Ami's story clearly illustrates, patients we can refuse to take on the role imposed on them by the doctor's or parent's metaphors, and insist on their own as the leading metaphor for the situation. Ami never used the martial metaphor so pervasive in the cultural discourse around illness. He didn't talk about "killing pain," as he didn't see pain as a passive happening inflicted on him as a helpless victim. And the metaphorical flexibility encouraged by Isaac generated a rich enough mixture of metaphors with which all three participants--patient, parent and physician--could interpret reality.

Language is a design for living, Postman says. To talk is to imagine a world of make-believe, to hypothesize that everything is like something else. During one of Isaac's last visits with Ami, who was increasingly losing the ability to breathe, Ami demanded to know what would happen next. Isaac explained that were he to stop breathing, he may have to be intubated by tracheotomy and helped to breathe mechanically. Ami understood he didn't need that yet, but that the day was nearing, and he wanted to make sure Isaac understood he wanted it. Completely dependent on the people around him, at the weight of a child of five, his words barely uttered, and discerned with great difficulty, he wanted to live. His narrative was one of passion for life. His metaphor: carpe diem or seize the day.

ROCKING HASSAN: AVOIDING DEFINITION TYRANNY

In a chapter titled "Definition Tyranny," Postman (1976) explains that in every situation, someone or some group has a decisive power of definition. To have power means to be able to define and to make the definition stick. He adds further that there's no escaping the jurisdiction of definitions, and that social order requires that there be established definitions (sometimes fixed and formal, sometimes fluid and informal).

There is no system without official definitions and authoritative sources to enforce them. However, an enhanced sensibility to semantic environments and their language provides us with the capacity to maintain a certain psychological distance from conventional definitions. And this is a valuable asset. To have to speak someone else's words, to have our own attitudes governed by someone else's definitions, can be a very dangerous situation. And this is what Postman calls Definition Tyranny.

To avoid definition tyranny it is useful to ask questions such as who or what is the source of the definition; what is the source of his or her authority; is it economic power?; the Law?; Or is it knowledge? We should also ask ourselves to what extent we participated in granting the authority; what attitude towards us and others is promoted by the definition and to what extent can we play a role in changing the definition.

Policy reflects the ideology, conceptions and definitions of the policy-makers of the central ideas and issues in any given field. In the area of healthcare generally and in the context of hospital policies specifically, one of the issues that has received attention in the past years is the issue of visiting hours. Policies regarding visiting hours reflect hospitals' definitions of what families are and their conceptions of the competence of parents in situations of illness of their children. Family-centered policies reflect a set of values, attitudes, and approaches to the medical treatment of children that recognize that the family is the constant in the child's life, and that parents are the experts on the child's abilities and needs. These policies' focus is not only on the biomedical aspects of a child's condition but also on the child as a whole.

Hospitalized children lie in their beds facing fearful illness; surrounded by overwhelming noise from pulsating ventilators and monitors; invaded by the nurses' ministrations and overhearing strange and scary conversations. And all of this is aggravated by their being alone. Some hospitals have understood how traumatic this situation is and have liberalized their visiting hour policies. In some hospitals the changes have been revolutionary and there are now 24 hour visitation policies, or rooming-in as it is sometimes known. This has been found to be mostly beneficial and created only moderate discomfort to the staff. The presence of the parent improves the child's emotional state generally and, in anxiety provoking situations such as invasive tests, where not only the presence but the participation of the parent are encouraged, have even been shown to improve medical outcomes.

In 1977, the policy of the Chief of Pediatrics at the hospital where Isaac began to work that year was one of extreme limitations. The parents were literally allowed to only "visit" their children one hour a day. This stemmed from a conception or narrative in which parents are thought of as incompetent and a nuisance and interference with treatment.

Having just arrived in Israel and new to the hospital, Isaac went for his first visit to the baby ward. There--among all the other babies--he saw Hassan, a 9 month old baby, who was suffering of profound malnutrition.

The treatment and nutrition being given to Hassan was not working, and so Isaac decided to "adopt" the baby. Isaac picked Hassan up, held him in his arms, and went for long walks back and forth along the ward corridors every opportunity he got, a few times every day. Hassan began to gain weight, then he started to smile too, and six weeks later he was strong and healthy enough to be released from the hospital. Isaac continued to see him periodically and to follow Hassan's development as an outpatient for the following year.

It is, of course, not suggested here that it was Isaac's actions exclusively that made Hassan better. But his understanding of the power of definitions and his symbolic response to the policies and rules of the department allowed him to add to the baby's treatment the time-old medicine of TLC (Tender Loving Care) that is known to have a great effect on patients--adults and children.

Isaac did not break the rules. As a new immigrant in the country and a new doctor in the hospital, his courage did not go that far. But he avoided definition tyranny by refusing to respond to the rules the way they are designed to make us respond-- with blind obedience. He refused to fall prey to the propaganda inherent in every institution's policies and definitions.

Propaganda is used here not as it refers to the goodness or badness of the causes of hospital administrators, but as language as it is used in the implementation of policy; language that asks us "to believe" and not "to consider" and is designed to evoke a particular kind of response from doctors, nurses and families of patients: the automatic, immediate response of blind compliance.

As opposed to symbolic reactions that are reflective, delayed and mindful, signal responses are reflexive, immediate, kneejerk responses .What Isaac did was follow the General Semantics edict and took control of his reaction: he refused to be tyrannized by the boss's definitions, and found a way to put some distance between him and "the system's" way of defining things. In the absence of parents, Isaac redefined Hassan so that he was not only a patient but a baby far from his parents, and he redefined his job to include some of what are usually regarded as responsibilities of families or relatives.

By controlling or delaying his response, by providing his own definition to policy, he refused to be controlled by the complex Jacques Ellul (1964) called "La technique," the complex or semantic environment of the hospital that includes many additional means through which human behavior is organized and controlled: the life-sustaining, beeping machines in the hospital, insurance policies, HMO's, Electronic Health Records, 12 minute visits, etc. It is an environment that so many doctors and especially administrators have become so highly committed to, that it seems to have come to overshadow all other considerations.

In 1997, Isaac became ill and was hospitalized in the same hospital where he worked. One morning, while being rolled in his wheelchair to have a test done, a middle-aged man approached him. He greeted Isaac, wished him good health and walked away. That afternoon, a young man of 21 appeared in Isaac's room, a box of chocolates in his hand. He stood next to Isaac's bed and said: "My name is Hassan, do you remember me? My father told me you were sick. I just came to wish you a fast recovery and lots of health."

This is a story about conflicting narratives; about the gap between the definitions of an organization that is ruled by methods, and the human behavior of one doctor who refused to be controlled by them.

Hassan was told by his father the story of how Isaac had treated him, and incorporated into his life-narrative generally or he wouldn't have gone through the trouble of coming to visit and "return the favor." Just as it couldn't be claimed that Isaac's walks with Hassan in his arms were what made Hassan better, it is hard to claim that Hassan's visit made Isaac healthy. But the event left him gratified and elated, and it was a confirmation of his narrative. This was time-binding--the distinctively human attribute of preserving memories and records of experiences for the use of subsequent generations; the idea that progress is made by the fact that each generation adds to the material and spiritual wealth which it inherits.

A Good Question: Dalia's Mom and the Extensional Orientation

General Semantics encourages us to adopt an "extensional orientation" or to focus, as much as possible, on "factual information" and not on our subjective world-view that relies on abstract and general verbal definitions ("intensional orientation").

An extensional approach or orientation is neutral and factual. It requires of us the suspension of judgment, objective gathering and analysis of facts, and continual reality–testing.

As Johnson (1947) explains, achieving an extensional orientation requires us to conduct our questioning and answering habits in a scientific manner: to ask clear, answerable questions in a calm and unprejudiced manner and to revise any beliefs or assumptions that we held before in light of the answers obtained. This allows us to keep our information, beliefs, and theories up to date and to change our mind sufficiently often. This is important for everyone, whether the problems involved are classified as technical, ethical, political, or of course, medical.

Dalia suffered of rheumatoid arthritis, required very close attention and came to visit Isaac frequently, especially in the early stages of the development of the illness, always accompanied by her mother.

Every time Dalia and her mother came to Isaac, he examined Dalia and then sat down to talk to both of them. Since the age of the child allowed for it, Isaac's approach was to begin by asking Dalia to tell the story of her illness in her own words and allowed her to share what she perceived as relevant and reveal her personal views on her experiences since their last visit. Then he turned to the mother and asked her to describe her own views and elaborate on details. Dalia's narrative as well as her mother's included only very general comments about their daily life and relationships at home.

On one occasion, after Isaac finished Dalia's examination, and talking to the child first and then the mother about the development of the disease and planning for what instructions to provide about the treatment, Isaac simply asked the mother: "And how are you?" Tears filled the mother's eyes at the sound of the question and Isaac did not have to say almost anything more for the remainder of the conversation. The question had been enough for the mother to open up and go into a long narrative describing the difficulties she had been experiencing lately as a result of the attention she needed to give to Dalia. She also described at great length and detail how the jealousy of the younger siblings at home was making everything even harder and more complex, and how her husband--Dalia's father-- could not be counted on to cooperate and help.

As Postman (1976) says, all answers we ever get are responses to questions. The questions may not be evident to us, but they are nonetheless doing their work--to design the form that our knowledge will take and therefore to determine the direction of our actions.

The type of words used in a question determines the type of words used in the answer. Vague questions, for example, lead to vague answers, and this can lead to frustration. But the vague and general question "How are you?"--with the emphasis on the word "you"-- worked well in this case thanks to its timing. In other words, very open questions such as "how are you?" are questions that doctors, like all other people, ask in an automatic way, usually when first greeting their patients and their parents as they enter the room. They are the kinds of question that seem to not have anything to do with the medical context specifically. However, when asked some time into the meeting, after hearing only about the child and her illness, its transparency disappeared and it was charged with a very different meaning. It focused attention on the mother and conveyed to her the message that the physician was interested in how she was coping, too.

The high level of abstraction of its wording--that often times means questions are unanswerable--in this case helped Dalia's mother provide a detailed, low-abstraction answer. Also, the question did not have the structural or grammatical characteristics of questions that ask for either-or answers, for example. Isaac did not ask "And are you OK?" He had a feeling she wasn't, but was careful to pay attention to the assumptions that were underlying his question--to subject his assumption to scrutiny--and to ask it in a more open way.

Asking open-ended questions and allowing parents to talk openly can help in soliciting information on even the most sensitive topics. An open, nonjudgmental tone reassures both children and parents that the physician is interested and willing to discuss any topic. Moreover, in pediatrics, parents may not be able to put into words or ask themselves, what it is that scares them the most about their child's condition. Open ended questions allow for the parents' concerns to come to the surface.

It did not come as a surprise to Isaac that starting that day Dalia began to respond better to the treatment. Not a lot was said by Isaac in that conversation, but hidden behind the doctor's question "How are you?" was a test of his assumption that part of the problem was that Dalia's mom had not made her "side of the story" heard. She had kept her own, personal narrative out of view and to herself, and regarded it as illegitimate. The question released the narrative, allowed the mother her own voice, thus alleviating some of the tension that was interfering with life at home and with Dalia's treatment.

Rude Awakening: Mystification, Role Fixation and Dating

It was Isaac's first year of practice of pediatrics after four years of training. A young woman holding a two week old baby came into his office. The baby seemed generally healthy but he had been born with a cleft lip and palate. After examining the baby, evaluating her condition, and providing advice to the mother about feeding techniques, he referred the mother to a plastic surgeon. The mother dressed the baby, picked up her bags, thanked the doctor and left the clinic. As Isaac later found out, the baby underwent surgery and the cleft palate and lip were fixed.

About a year later, as the neonatologist on call at the hospital, Isaac was called to attend to the birth of the same woman's second child. The baby seemed to be in distress. It was a complicated birth that required suction and oxygen by mask, but the thorough examination found him to be well.

About a month later, the mother brought her baby for a check-up at Isaac's office. The doctor examined the baby and then sat down to discuss his care with the mother. All was well. It was a routine visit and there were no unusual or problematic issues to discuss. Isaac asked questions, listened to the mother's concerns, asked how the older girl was doing and what their home routine was like with two little babies at home. And before concluding the visit, he asked whether there was anything else she would like to say or ask.

Obviously surprised, her bags all packed and on her lap, her whole demeanor--one of someone who thought the visit was over and was beginning to move in the direction of the door--the mother took a deep breath, and obviously debating within herself whether she should say what she was thinking or not, she finally said softly: "Dr. Berger, where were you all this time?" Not understanding exactly what she meant, he asked her to explain, upon which she went into a long monologue about how Isaac's examinations had been thorough and his instructions helpful with both of her children, but that his attitude had changed completely and he now showed great involvement and empathy. And that this was not the case the first time around.

Surprised and embarrassed, Isaac wanted to ask the mother to put her bag down and talk to him some more. But he couldn't. He just said he was sorry and closed the door behind the mother, needing a few minutes before he could call the next patient in.

She was right. He could actually envision himself and remember his very professional, matter-of-fact demeanor just a few months back. He had no idea when this had changed and when he felt sure enough of himself to let go of his aloof and removed attitude. But the mother's remarks had forced him to think about it. She said he had been cold and unsympathetic, and she emphasized that the most maddening part of it was that he seemed to insist on using words that she couldn't understand and that left her more confused than before, and with more questions than answers.

A young doctor still, arrogant (as doctors can be, especially when they can first attach the letters M.D. to their names) mostly out of insecurity, this was clearly mystification.

Mystification, as Postman (1976) defines it, is a process whereby ideas or events which are perfectly understandable to almost anybody, are talked about in a way that is inaccessible to all but a select group of people. A cleft palate and lip are a condition that can be easily explained to parents of babies born with the condition. But as it happens in other professions, doctors too, sometimes use their technical vocabularies to indicate exclusiveness or linguistic elitism. But when this happens with doctors, and especially with pediatricians, the consequences can be very serious, as parents (the laypersons in the semantic environment) must know exactly what is going on and understand the doctors' instructions, but also feel like the person to whom they have entrusted their children's health and wellbeing, actually cares about them. What doctors achieve in their insistence on using polysyllabic technical terms to denote commonplace and easily curable disorders, or even the more complicated ones, is the mystification of their patients who leave their clinics terrified.

The mother's words were a rude awakening for Isaac. But there was a positive or optimistic side to the story. He had changed and not committed what is known in General Semantics as role fixation, and not fallen in love with the self he had created through his use of language when the first baby was born.

Quoting George Herbert Mead, Postman (1976) explains that all selves are called into existence by social context, and that there's no existence except as we exist in a situation. For all practical purposes, he adds, what we are is how we conduct ourselves in different environments, and our conduct is predominantly language. The language we use elicits a certain kind of response from others. Isaac's language as the self he was while caring for the first baby elicited pain and insult from the mother, while the language he used as the second self he became just a year later, elicited trust and openness. The language in this particular semantic environment produced consequences which he did not anticipate. The mother made him realize that, thankfully, he had not gotten stuck in the first self and its way of talking, which happens sometimes because in the situation where it is appropriate, it works well for us.

"We feel competent in that role," Postman says,

> ...and therefore feel confident that we can control the situation. Our hypotheses about the responses of others are confirmed...But we run into difficulty when we enter situations in which our favorite role is not appropriate. (p. 116)

People who cannot transit from one semantic environment to another are "role-fixated." Doctors need to develop semantic flexibility--the ability to move with competence through a wide range of semantic environments in their encounters with different patients. And patients, on their part, need to understand the General Semantics concept of "dating."

"Dating" is the term used in General Semantics to describe the process of attaching dates to our evaluations to remind ourselves of changes occurring over time. The idea is that if our evaluations and our statements about our environment are to be accurate, they must take into consideration the fact that both humans and their environments change from moment to moment.

A Doctor in 2000 is not the same Doctor in 2014. For Isaac, this was made clear by the two babies' mother even in the span of just one year: Isaac1961 was not the same as Isaac1962.

GOOD LION, BAD LION: SELF-REFLEXIVE NIGHTMARES

Dani was a charming five year old. He was communicative, friendly and healthy all-around. He had been a good sleeper since birth but when he came in with his father one day, he seemed sad and his father, exhausted.

Isaac had barely said, "Hello," they had just sat down across from him and the father had already made it very clear why they had come to see the doctor: Dani wasn't sleeping well and, as a result, neither was the rest of the family.

There was a pattern. Dani was put to bed every night at around 8 pm and fell asleep easily, but for the past month or so he was waking up 2-3 times every night crying and screaming. At first, the parents came in to his bedroom, consoled him for a few minutes, and went back to bed. On the second night they took his temperature and found out he did not have a fever. They brought him a glass of water, and caressed him for a while. By the second week the parents were taking turns sitting next to Dani and helping him back to sleep a few times a night. And they were getting worried. Trying not to have the entire household awake for the whole night, they did not go into long conversations with Dani at night. They talked to him over breakfast, attempting to understand from him what it was that was bothering him, to no avail. The only reply they were getting to their guiding questions was a shy "I don't know."

The parents had, by this point, developed a complex theory. They had made an appointment to talk to Dani's kindergarten teacher and asked her about Dani's behavior: Was he playing with his friends? Had any of the kids made fun of him? Were the teachers paying attention to him? They had spoken to Dani's babysitter, suspecting she was mistreating him. By the third week they were scared and exhausted, and the tension was getting the best of them. The parents were arguing and fighting all the time.

The process was self-reflexive. They were spiraling and making things worse by the language they were using to try to explain their son's lack of sleep.

Language is self-reflexive. As Korzybski (1958) described it, using language is like being in a mirrored room. Dani's parents had moved very fast from the low level of abstraction that was the fact that Dani was waking up in the middle of the night, to the high level of abstraction where they thought perhaps someone was abusing their child or that there was a very serious problem underlying his lack of sleep. Their fears that their entire family life would be disrupted had become a self-fulfilling prophecy as they were constantly tired, worried, having trouble functioning at work, and projecting their concerns onto Dani during the day. They had made a prediction that was coming true because they had made the prediction.

Isaac listened to the father quietly for a while and then turned to Dani. Aware of how nonverbal communication can automatically enhance the relationship with the child, he positioned himself so that he was looking at Dani directly at eye level rather than standing and towering over him. And he simply asked: "Who wakes you up every night?" To which Dani immediately replied: "A bad lion scares me. He wants to swallow me."

Apparently uncomfortable about how quickly Isaac had gotten an answer from Dani, the father immediately interjected that Dani had mentioned a lion, and that they had explained to him that the lion did not exist and that it was only a dream, but that it hadn't helped.

Isaac faced Dani again, smiled at him and pulled out of his left side desk drawer a little stuffed toy lion. Holding it away from Dani, waiting to see his reaction, Isaac said: "I am going to help you. Starting tonight, you can go to sleep holding this lion. I have told the lion that his job is to protect you and chase away the bad lion every time he comes around. This lion is very strong. So you will be able to sleep well if he is with you every night." Dani didn't smile. But he reached for the toy, and by the time they left the office he was holding it tight.

Five days later, Dani's father called to report that Dani was still waking up at night but was falling asleep within minutes and that for the last two nights they hadn't even had to come into his room.

Self-reflexiveness is a semantic process by which we try to order and control our world. The parents had started generating expectations because this was their way of preparing themselves for what would happen to them. But their world had started to become even more disorganized and unpredictable as they were not aware of what they were doing and how they were doing it. They were creating what they had expected.

Isaac did not point out to the father that this is what he and Dani's mother were doing. But the doctor had stopped the spiral first, by building a relationship not only with the parent but also with the patient. The point was to not only collect data, but to build a relationship in which both Dani and his father felt respected, supported, and trusting. And he did this by seeing the child and listening to him. By showing him he was really interested in him and turning him into an active participant in his own care.

But he did more than that. He paid attention to the degree of specificity of Dani's utterances. These were low in abstraction, and so they denoted the color and texture and uniqueness of what was bothering him. This allowed Isaac to descend even further on the ladder of abstraction--all the way down to the non-verbal level where he found the toy lion. And then he called the toy "a good lion."

Things do not have real names, but things and the names we give them are hard to separate. What we call things affects how we perceive them. We identify names and words with things. And so, if we change the names of things, we change how people regard them, and this is as good as changing the nature of the thing itself--in this case--the dream.

Isaac had generated a new and useful way of perceiving the lion in the dream--a new perspective on it. He had altered the imagery and by doing so, he had dissipated the fears. Perceiving the problem from various level of abstraction, he had used both first and second-order thinking: He first worked within the framework of Dani's world, accepting the assumptions on which it was based (first order). But he then went outside the frame of the problem, and drawing on resources not contained in the original frame, suggested an alternative narrative (second order). By changing the words--or in this case adding a good lion to the bad--he reframed the problem and found a solution.

By the time Dani came back for his next visit, there were no more bad dreams. He had started the first grade. Isaac and Dani talked about school, about Dani's teachers and his friends, his birthday party and a recent soccer game.

I AM THE PATIENT: TIME-BINDING THE TRANSITION FROM CHILDHOOD TO YOUNG ADULTHOOD

In part I we discussed the idea of time-binding, the General Semantics term that refers to what characterizes us as humans due to our unique capacity to connect and integrate the past, the present and the future, thanks to language and symbolic communication

All of the stories here are stories of time-binding--stories of the therapeutic activities created by Isaac for and with his patients over time, helping them maintain a sense of continuity and stability amidst change. But the current story is rooted completely in the idea of time-binding.

The importance of continuity became especially clear to Isaac when, on one occasion, many years ago, he was summoned for a house call. Bag in hand, he rang the bell. A young woman opened the door and let him in. They exchanged greetings, she offered Isaac a glass of water, and invited him to sit down in the living room.

Feeling increasingly awkward about the length of the initial encounter and wanting to get to the point, Isaac asked could she now take him to the patient. A bit blushed and obviously embarrassed, the woman said: "I am the patient."

Recovering from the surprise, Isaac asked to go back to the beginning. As it turned out, this was Anat, whom Isaac had not seen in a few years. His secretary had written down the name and address but it hadn't sounded familiar. Anat had been his patient since she was a baby, and he had followed her development and managed her diabetes for years, until she went away to college. Her treatment had been balanced and she was thriving, doing well in school and enjoying every minute of it.

Anat was now home for the holidays, and for the first time in a long time, her insulin levels were out of balance. The thought of calling another doctor hadn't even crossed her mind.

Transitioning from their teenage years to adulthood can be stressful for kids with diabetes and their families. Teens and young adults find themselves needing to assume more responsibility for the management of their illness and to make more independent judgments about their health care needs. And many of them find it very hard to transition from their pediatrician to a different physician.

Teens with special needs or chronic health problems and their parents are especially reluctant to leave a pediatrician they've been comfortable with for years, but they are not the only ones. The issue of when the right time is for this transition is a central topic in health care generally today. Every kid outgrows the pediatrician at some point—but when that point comes can vary. Some patients can't wait to escape the colorful band-aids, the little chairs and the fluffy clouds on the walls, whereas others feel uncomfortable being the youngest patients in the grown-up internist's waiting room, along with men and women 30 and 40 years their elders.

More and more young adults are choosing to stay with their pediatricians at least through their college years. Even though most colleges have health services on campus, when students are home for weekends and holidays and need a doctor, the pediatrician's office seems like the only option to them. It feels to them like the most natural choice to call the physician they have known all their lives.

This trend has become so common, that many pediatric practices are making sure their offices are comfortable for older teens with, for example, separate waiting areas and different reading material, and of course, adolescent specialists on staff. And some major medical centers have even opened young-adult clinics to help ease the transition. And there is even a growing medical specialty known as "med-peds"--for doctors certified in both internal medicine and pediatrics--which is also helping provide more continuity.

Similarly to the stage when childhood, as Postman (1982) explains, began to be understood as a social category and a psychological condition in the sixteenth century as an outgrowth of literacy, so adolescence emerged as a clearly separate social and psychological category 30 or 40 years ago as a result, among other factors, of changes in the media environment. And so young adulthood is now beginning to be conceptualized as a separate and special category, with many health risks and behaviors with potentially lasting effects, such as sexually transmitted diseases, eating disorders, substance abuse and mental-health issues that are a result of various factors such puberty coming earlier than ever in both boys and girls, research breakthroughs extending the life span of sufferers of certain disease , the sociology of the millennials and the economy.

In the U.S., the economic factor includes, for example, the fact that many young adults often fall into a medical void after they leave their pediatrician and don't have a primary-care doctor until their 30s or 40s, and this is the source of much worry among health-care experts. The new health-reform bill, that allows dependents to stay on their parents' insurance plans until age 26, helps narrow this health-care gap for young adults. And from the point of view of medical breakthroughs and discoveries, for example, more patients are living longer with chronic illnesses like cystic fibrosis or autism. Being able to continue taking care of such patients all the way through adulthood provides a blessed continuity.

Whether their patients leave at age18 or 21, or they feel comfortable seeing the doctor who treated their diaper rash well into their 20's, pediatricians are the ultimate time-binding doctors. They are often their patients' life-long companions and advisors. They form bonds with them that last into young adulthood and sometimes beyond. Like other pediatricians, Isaac draws the line when patients become parents themselves. But the relationship continues as they then often start coming in to see him with their own children.

QUINTUPLETS AND INDEXING: BABY1 IS NOT BABY2 IS NOT BABY3 IS NOT BABY4 IS NOT BABY5

The great advances in technological developments in the field of in-vitro fertilization have dramatically increased the number of multiple births throughout the world over the past three decades or so, and this has been the case especially in Israel.

The world's first IVF baby was born in the UK in 1979, and just four years later, Israel's first IVF baby followed. Since then, Israel has become a world-leader in IVF treatment. Israel has multiple recognized fertility centers--more fertility clinics per capita than any other nation--and it also has the highest per capita rate of IVF procedures. In Israel, both married and single women up to the age of 45, are permitted virtually unlimited IVF attempts, and not just for a first baby, but for subsequent babies, too. Women from age 45 to 51 are permitted to continue treatments with donated ova, and there are no waiting lists. The State of Israel provides health care along the continuum from family planning services through childbirth, and much of reproductive care is funded by the government and through health funds.

This reproductive care policy reflects Jewish religious, cultural, and social norms regarding fertility. Parenthood is considered a basic human right based on biblical and other Jewish religious sources. Beginning with the verse "...and God said unto them, be fruitful and multiply, and replenish the earth, and subdue it" (Genesis 1:28), and all the way to the policies of the State of Israel in modern times, the personal desire for parenthood, and especially motherhood, has been ingrained in Jewish culture, strengthened further by the historical persecution of Jews in the Diaspora, the Holocaust, and the continuing loss of life in Arab-Israeli wars and terrorist acts. And a person's right to procreate (especially the superior right to motherhood), have been recognized in Supreme Court rulings (as opposed to the right to choose abortion). This combination of reproductive technology, religion, culture, ideology and policy, has led to an increased incidence of multiple births in the country.

Close to 30 years ago, quintuplets were born in the city of the hospital where Isaac worked. As the senior neonatologist at the hospital, Isaac was the chief physician in charge of the new babies, beginning with his presence in the delivery room, throughout their prolonged stay in the premature nursery, and all the way through their discharge at about 10 weeks of age, with an array of instructions, and follow-ups at the outpatient clinic for the first year.

As part of Israel's socialized medicine system, part of which is still in place today, Well Baby Care is provided to all babies in the community. Physicals, measurements, immunizations, feeding guidance and development follow-ups, are all done in clinics located in almost every neighborhood.

Understanding how complicated the logistics would be to get even to the corner clinic with the five babies--who also had an older sister--and trying to make sure that the Well Baby Care was performed on time, Isaac arranged to make an exception and to conduct home visits himself, as well as to have a nurse visit the family periodically to perform all the necessary care for the babies, and provide advice for their parents at least during the babies' first year of life.

After the first year elapsed, the mother called Isaac and let him know that they had talked about it and they had decided to continue their care at Isaac's afternoon private clinic. When Isaac asked if they were sure this is what they would like, since there were other, perhaps more convenient, possibilities, the woman replied that they were absolutely sure, and explained that they had known this for a very long time, since the babies were in the incubators months before. Many healthcare professionals had come in touch with them and treated their babies through very trying times. They had all been very professional and some of them even nice and empathetic. But Isaac had been the only one to talk to them about their babies using their names and not referring to them as "the quintuplets" or "the babies."

Isaac was touched. It was clear to him that a special effort was necessary, based on the sheer number of the babies, to not forget that each of them was a separate individual. And he made the effort.

As General Semantics teaches us, our tendency is to think of the world in categories, and to disregard the differences among the individuals who make up each category. Perhaps the periodic house calls helped this process in later stages, as Isaac got to know the five babies not in the environment of the hospital or clinic, but in the context of each of their corners, rooms, and favorite places at home. But his insistence on learning their names, talking to them and about them using these names, and connecting them as he would do with every other little patient with their little faces, began at the hospital, when they were just a few weeks old, weighing less than one kilogram each. From the very beginning, Isaac insisted on indexing: remembering that baby1 is not baby2 is not baby3 is not baby4 is not baby5; that they are not "the babies" and not "the quintuplets" but Orli, Shai, Tom, Adina and Michal.

The literature on the psychology of multiple birth babies is very vast. It discusses an array of issues including personality and the complexity of identity; family relationships; the babies' social and emotional development and its effect on their progress in school; language development, etc. But not nearly enough attention is paid in it to the importance of indexing.

As the children grew, the parents began to come for visits and checkups with each of the kids separately. They were never dressed in similar outfits, they were encouraged to develop their separate interests, and as hard as it was, they were dedicated one-on-one time. And they were each praised or punished individually.

Isaac became a partner in the parents' hard work to establish their children's individual identities. They would forever share a birthday and a very special bond, but they would each have their own thoughts and feelings, likes and dislikes. And Isaac was intent on fostering their individuality from day one. They kept coming to see him throughout the years. He watched them grow and develop and turn into wonderful adults. Their mutual affection grew, and the trust the parents had put on Isaac endured. On occasion, he is consulted on the health of the next generation: Orli's girls, Tom's twins, or Shai's baby boy.

MY BAR MITZVAH GIFT: BEHAVIOR, EXPERIENCE AND BY-PASSING

The main principle of the transactional perspective on communication is that all perception and all experience is a transaction. The nature of a transaction is such that the two parties involved are both shaped by their relationship with each other. Neither party is ever passive or simply acted-on.

The idea, expressed in various ways to this point, is that people do not exist independently from the situation they are in. And that these situations are transactions.

Transactions imply two actors, and not someone who is an actor and someone else who is "acted-upon." In other words, the roles that participants play in any situation define each other. The batter defines the pitcher and vice versa, the seller defines the buyer and vice versa, and so it is with the teacher and the learner and, of course, with the doctor and the patient. The doctor does not act upon the patient. The patient is an active participant in the situation, whose role shapes that of the physician, as Isaac would learn very early on in his pediatric career.

In 1964, on his last year of pediatric residency at Michael Reese Hospital in Chicago, Isaac learned a great lesson from Jack, a 13 year old boy suffering from leukemia.

Jack spent many weeks at a time in the hospital, a significant part of that time in isolation, to protect him from infections. He was an introverted, thin youngster. He seemed frail and very sad.

The doctor-patient relationship was generally good. For anyone on the outside looking in at their encounters, the relationship would seem professional, civilized and correct. It was clear Jack liked Isaac, as at some point he asked for him to be the doctor who performs the necessary procedures, tests, treatments and transfusions. But Jack's distant demeanor and what Isaac inferred as the boy's need for privacy and space, or his shyness, made Isaac refrain from making much conversation, or from asking questions about his feelings beyond the physical ones. This was hard for Isaac. He was, from very early on in his practice, a believer in the healing power of communication and in emotional bonds with patients as part of the processes of healing and coping. But it was just as well, as the Chief of Pediatrics had called him to let him know that if he didn't take a step back, he would be taken off various cases. To be a good doctor, the boss said, there needed to be objectivity and detachment.

As it turned out, this is not what Jack wanted. He really liked Isaac. He trusted him and kept hoping that he would spend some more time with him. He wished he could talk to him about his life and not only about his illness – about who he was in his own eyes and not only in the context of the hospital and his medical treatment. But Isaac didn't know this and he read Jack's gestures, tone and body language as further proof that a comforting smile and very matter-of-fact exchanges were what was right for the patient. At least until Jack did something that stopped the spiral of wrong inferences.

On a cold winter day, while on his morning rounds, Isaac walked in to Jack's room. He greeted him, asked how he was feeling and was there anything unusual this morning. In his usual quiet way Jack replied briefly, mostly with yes or no. Isaac examined him and while drawing blood for a few necessary tests, Jack said: "You have to congratulate me, today is my bar mitzvah." Surprised at the unusual personal character of the utterance, Isaac smiled, and congratulated Jack warmly. They talked for a few more minutes and getting up to leave the room, Isaac said "mazel tov" and wished Jack health. "Dr. Berger," said Jack, "before you go, could you please open the closet and hand me the box on the shelf?" Isaac complied and handed Jack the small package. "This is my Bar Mitzvah gift" said Jack. "Oh, how nice" said Isaac and added: "what did you get?" "No" replied Jack: "This is my Bar Mitzvah present for you."

Isaac had just learned a lesson – that much was clear. But he wasn't sure then what the lesson was. He just knew he had been deeply moved. His face blushed and his eyes filled with tears. He held Jack's hand, thanked him, and promised to return to see him that afternoon.

It was a lesson in gratitude of course, but more importantly, it was a lesson on the difference between behavior and experience, about the difficulty of inferring the latter from the former, and about by-passing.

British psychiatrist R. D. Laing (1966) talked about the process of perception in communication. His theory is that one's communicative behavior is largely shaped by one's perception (or experience) of the relationship with the person we are communicating with.

Laing made a distinction between experience and behavior. Behavior is the observable actions of another. It is public. Experience, on the other hand, is private. It is the feeling that accompanies behavior, or the perception of another's behavior. And it consists of the imagination of the future, the perception of the present and the memory of the past. Experiences are internal and they are not accessible to anyone else. They cannot be observed.

And so, at the heart of human communication is the process of inferring experience from behavior. This is a hard process, as Isaac found out. When interacting with Jack, he had two levels of experience: his direct perspective of Jack, but also his experience of Jack's experience. This is what Laing called "meta-perspective": our inference that what we imagine others are thinking or feeling is what they are actually feeling. In Jack's case, Isaac's inference was wrong. He was yearning for a closer relationship and for communication about more than leukemia. Our meta-perspectives may or may not be accurate and when they are not, misunderstandings happen. Isaac had assumed a great deal of what he thought he knew about Jack. He had been meta-perceiving--inferring from Jack's behavior what his experience was of the illness, the hospital and their relationship.

By-passing is the act of responding to words as if their meaning was in them--in the words--and not in the people using them and, thus, as if they mean the same thing to different people. There were not many words in these doctor and patient encounters at first aside from the most basic and functional ones. But the physician took the same kind of risk taken when we by-pass what people mean by words and assumed understanding based on his interpretation of the patient's non-verbal cues.

For the most part, we do not get our perceptions from "out there." Our perceptions come from within us. We see things not as they are but as we are. And we do not change our perception on the basis of verbal information alone, but through acting on our perceptions and encountering hitches which require us to modify our perceptions. Jack modified Isaac's perception of him with the beautiful gesture of giving Isaac a gift on the occasion of his own bar mitzvah. He was not the sad and remote child Isaac thought he was, generally, and he wasn't sad all the time, either. And he definitely wasn't fragile. He was optimistic, he had a positive outlook on life, and was determined to get better.

CHAPTER 5
Doctoring as a Subversive Activity

———■———

Among the essential traits a physician should have is
interest in people, because the secret of curing is caring.
—Dr. Francis Peabody

IT HAS BEEN 10 YEARS since Isaac retired. He does not work at a hospital anymore, but he still sees patients at a child development center and in his private practice. In the course of these few years since his official retirement, the world of medicine has seen many developments in both medical research and healthcare related technology.

A quick look at the major trends in health and medicine reveals innumerable discoveries that are bringing about cures to illnesses previously regarded as incurable. There are developments in cancer immunotherapy, for example, that are finding ways to overcome some of the problems of conventional chemotherapy such as the fact that currently available compounds kill normal cells as well as cancer cells, leading to serious side effects.

There are also data-rich wearable devices and sensors. Among these are, for example, wearable heart rate monitors that don't just mimic the look of an EKG, but also collect clinically usable data on heart signals. There are open platforms that integrate the data from patients' devices directly into their electronic health records. Patients with insulin-dependent diabetes, for example, can now use an app to aggregate glucometer, insulin pump and continuous blood glucose monitor data, and transmit it to their providers via the platform.

Great emphasis is put also on developing technologies to aid health communication. Some of the trends here include the increasing role of social media in health care, which is said to lead to empowered, engaged and better informed patients. Patients are indeed going online for health related information, to share their experiences and find support. And doctors too are using social media for professional purposes. Social media offer opportunities to promote public health, improve health delivery and at some level at least, create productive relationships between patients and physicians. And they certainly provide companies with great marketing opportunities. There has been a growth in mobile marketing--health apps that can be used for medical and drug reference, to share EHR data, images, video and other resources with patients.

If one pays attention to the language used in the context of all of these developments, it is clear we have moved into an entirely new semantic environment. Just as in the civic realm the word "citizen" has almost entirely been replaced with the word "consumer," so in medicine the word "patient" is slowly being replaced by the word "client." People now talk about how the technology will allow us to "micro-target consumers when they are on the go and at other times when they are open to brand communications." One can also hear and read statements such as "the apps will give us a new way to build long-term relationships through offering high-value, client-focused content." And similar to the trends in other industries, in medicine too, the talk is less about patient satisfaction and increasingly about "measuring success," "initiatives translating into sales," "meaningful PR metrics" and "good relationships with health care brands."

In a world where patients are clients, it is only fit that doctors are called "medical providers." As Hartzband and Groopman (2011) explain,

The words "consumer" and "provider" are reductionist; they ignore the essential psychological, spiritual, and humanistic dimensions of the relationship--the aspects that traditionally made medicine a "calling," in which altruism overshadowed personal gain. Furthermore, the term "provider" is deliberately and strikingly generic, designating no specific role or type or level of expertise. Each medical professional--doctor, nurse, physical therapist, social worker, and more--has specialized training and skills that are not recognized by the all-purpose term "provider," which carries no resonance of professionalism...Rather, the generic term "provider" suggests that doctors and nurses and all other medical professionals are interchangeable. "Provider" also signals that care is fundamentally a prepackaged commodity on a shelf that is "provided" to the "consumer," rather than something personalized and dynamic, crafted by skilled professionals and tailored to the individual patient. (pp. 1372-1373)

Doctors are being harmed by the semantic epidemic, too. Very difficult demands are being placed on them by the system which is leading them to function below their level of personal excellence. They are caught in such an oppressive system, that many of them are choosing to abandon it. And many of those who remain in it are building walls of protection in the form of cynicism or detachment. In the process, they are losing that which used to be most precious to them: a sense of meaning and the opportunity to practice medicine in a way that is worthy of their dedication and love.

In a piece titled "Who Will Heal the Doctors?" that appeared in the *New York Times* on October 2nd, 2013, David Bornstein claims that the notion that a doctor is an objective scientist whose job is to come up with the one best solution to patients' problems is a view that is out of step with research on medical outcomes and much of what is known about the therapeutic aspects of the patient-doctor relationship. "People are not widgets" he says, and adds that medicine cannot be reduced to cutting and sewing or putting chemicals into the body. In the technological reality described above, more and more people are living with incurable diseases that would have killed them a in the past. And Bornstein explains:

> As the population ages, more health care will be directed to patients with chronic or terminal conditions. For doctors, care will become less a question of curing a disease than helping their patients to live as well as possible in the face of their illnesses. That's not the job they train you for in medical school. But in this emerging context, the doctor patient relationship becomes even more central. It may be the quality of this relationship that determines whether doctors can cope with, and derive satisfaction, from care that involves far less clinical certainty or control.

The semantic environment created by technology and bureaucracy has brought about an atmosphere in which it is only natural that the idea of evidence-based medicine will flourish. With all of its advantages and achievements, EBM has progressively left doctors without a choice but to focus their practice on the disease and not on the patient. They are led to consider a sick body or a sick part rather than a sick person, and they neglect the communicative and relational dimensions of their work. The language of Evidence

Based Medicine is the language of statistics which leaves out so many details that it is never about any patient in particular.

There is great hype over the technological innovations of the past few years, and some people are even questioning the future need for doctors at all. In an article that appeared in *The Atlantic* magazine on February 20th, 2013, Jonathan Cohn talks about IBM's Watson that has now been put to commercial use in a few hospitals. Watson is the same machine that beat Ken Jennings at *Jeopardy* and it is now, as Cohn puts it, "churning through case histories at Memorial Sloan-Kettering, learning to make diagnoses and treatment recommendations." He discusses just how far the automation of medicine might go, and the answer is quite clear from the title of the article: "The Robot Will See You Now."

Watson is not alone. Google Glass will soon be used in everyday healthcare, wellness or the so called "healthcare lifestyle" is being "gamified," there are new rules about direct-to-consumer genomics, and a 3D printer that can print artificial limbs and biomaterials, is soon to be mainstream. Home diagnostics are becoming more and more common, as are DIY biotechnologies. In other words, healthcare is being brought back to the home, but without the doctor, the side effect of which may be an epidemic of Semantic Iatrogenic Disease.

While the discourse around many of these developments is, paradoxically, all about bringing doctors and patients closer together, the names given to current and future medical technologies are very telling: they all point to the growing physical and psychological distance between them.

The technologies all fall under the general category of "telemedicine" which includes "robotic nurse assistants" for elderly patients in nursing homes and hospitals to perform basic medical procedures such as drawing blood; and "remote touch" technologies that will use the force-feedback technique used by the video-game industry. This of course, may reduce human error and improve what is known as "palpatory diagnosis" but it can never replace what we call palpatory empathy or the soothing that comes from a flesh and blood doctor's touch as she looks into our eyes. We know we are on the verge of a semantic iatrogenic epidemic when humanoid robots resembling the shape of the human body are discussed as eventually not only being able to provide basic care but keeping patients company as well.

In pediatrics specifically, new technologies include genomic sequencing helping clinicians obtain genetic diagnoses in acutely ill newborns or more timely diagnoses for children with behavioral disorders, an important development since neuroscientists have now confirmed that early intervention is crucial for children with behavioral and learning disorders. And there are even clinical trials of a blood test for autism based on "signatures" of gene activity. But along with these, there is also the raving about how humanoid robots will serve especially good companions for sick children.

These technological trends, combined with an atmosphere of confusion around the implications of the Affordable Care Act, commonly known as "Obamacare," have led to what Postman (1992) called Information Glut.

Without positioning ourselves on either side of the debate, it is clear that among all of its other implications, with the rising demands of a new dimension of healthcare delivery, where doctors need to see more patients to make up for lower reimbursement, Obamacare has raised the need to grapple with the changing image of the doctor, who has for a long time ceased to be the physician carrying a black bag and making house calls, and now communicates with patients and charges for consultation via text messages, e-mails and increasingly video chats, and prescribes, along with medication, internet sites as sources of information. Increasing attention is being paid to the measurement of physician efficiency in this new state of affairs, and it is predicted that physicians will be compensated based on their ability to effectively communicate with patients, and ensure patient compliance through these new media.

The Semantic Iatrogenic Disease is here. But the only way to stop it from becoming an epidemic, or at least keeping some of us safe from it, is for doctors to counter the technological and bureaucratic trends by insisting on playing the key role they always played in shaping the semantic medical environment; by looking at their doctoring as a subversive activity.

In their book titled *Teaching as a Subversive Activity*, Neil Postman and Charles Weingartner (1969) define subversive teaching as exposing students to those things they are not exposed to in culture. If what they are listening to outside of school is Madonna or Bruce Springsteen, for example, school should expose them to Mozart and Bach and Handel, they say.

To be subversive, teachers must encourage students to think beyond the conventional wisdom of popular culture. And to be subversive, doctors must think beyond the conventional wisdom of mainstream medicine and healthcare. Technological solutions to health problems will be available to patients. Apps, gadgets and internet platforms are here to stay. But along with their use of these technological innovations, doctors should channel their energies to the creation of a semantic environment that counters their iatrogenic side-effects. Doctors should aim at being the symphony to counter hypnotic, cataleptic Trance. They should, in Cassell's terms (1997) not only cure and heal, but "doctor," too. They should "be" and not just "do," and remember that they are not merely bearers of knowledge and skills in using tools and technologies, but are themselves the instruments of care.

If we insist on trying to fix all medical problems by using technology without paying attention to communication and relationships with patients, we turn healthcare into an institution that, as Postman and Weingartner (1969) put it in talking about schools, is inflicted on everybody. Their metaphor to describe the state of the educational system accurately describes what healthcare is doing, too:

> It is as if we are driving a multi-million-dollar sports car, screaming, "Faster! Faster!" while peering fixedly into the rear-view mirror... and it has been sheer dumb luck that we have not smashed ourselves to bits--so far. We have paid almost exclusive attention to the car, equipping it with all sorts of fantastic gadgets and an engine that will propel it at ever increasing speeds, but we seem to have forgotten where we wanted to go in it. (pp. 12-13)

As in other areas of life, constant, accelerating, ubiquitous change is the most central characteristic of the world of health and medicine. The abilities and attitudes required of doctors to deal adequately with change are of the highest priority and it is not beyond their ability to design a medical environment which can help patients heal and cope. If the institution we call "medicine" cures but doesn't heal, if it takes care of disease but induces alienation, it is not doing what it is meant to do. It must be changed. And it can be changed, through awareness of the concept of the semantic environment and the adoption of the tools of General Semantics.

This perspective has never been as urgent as now. Health reforms, economic limitations and technological developments have created an environment that requires physicians' subversion.

The same strategies suggested by various scholars and quoted by Postman and Weingartner (1969) in education are useful as tools of subversion in medicine. David Riesman would call it the "counter-cyclical" approach to medicine, meaning that doctors should stress values that are not stressed by the larger healthcare system. Norbert Wiener would insist that clinics now must function as "anti-entropic feedback systems" to slow down the tendency toward chaos. The process cannot be completely reversed but it can be slowed down and partly controlled. And one way to control it is through feedback.

As doctors are the ones to come in direct contact with patients, they must be the ones to recognize change, to be sensitive to problems caused by change, and to sound alarms when entropy accelerates to a dangerous degree. They must adopt an anthropological perspective that allows them to be part of their profession, of their system and their environment, and at the same time, to be out of it.

Achieving such a perspective is extremely difficult and requires of doctors the courage to free themselves of some of the system's constraints that have made them accustomed to a certain kind of talk and behavior. They must, for example, sensitize themselves to the unconscious effects of their habitual metaphors (from diagnoses such as sluggish cognitive tempo, to the metaphors reflected in visitation policies at hospitals, to the newer ones such as "remote touch") so they are not condemned to their constricted perceptions and can think of alternative modes of behavior and communication with their patients. As was illustrated in the stories of Isaac's patients, to curb the leading ideology of a system, physicians must recognize when their language--or the language of their group--is limited, misleading, or one-sided.

The developments in technology and policy in healthcare are not additive or linear but ecological. The field and the profession are not the way they were over 50 years ago when Isaac began to practice medicine. It is a totally new environment requiring a whole new repertoire of survival strategies for doctors as well as for their patients--new patterns of defense, perception, understanding, and evaluation. It is a new kind of medicine.

Norbert Wiener observed the paradox that results from our increasing technological capability in electronic communication and explained that as the number of messages increases, the amount of information carried decreases. The more media to communicate we have, the fewer significant ideas are communicated. Likewise, the more machines and tests, as well as EHR's and doctor-patient communication apps, the harder it becomes for doctors to listen to their patients and actually communicate with them.

Postman and Weingartner talk about what they call "the change revolution" and they illustrate what they mean, through the development of media of communication and the metaphor of a clock face.

> Imagine a clock face with sixty minutes on it. Let the clock stand for the time men have had access to writing systems. Our clock would thus represent something like three thousand years, and each minute on our clock fifty years. On this scale, there were no significant media changes until about nine minutes ago. At that time, the printing press came into use in Western culture. About three minutes ago, the telegraph, photograph, and locomotive arrived. Two minutes ago: the telephone, rotary press, motion pictures, automobile, aeroplane and radio. One minute ago, the talking picture. Television has appeared in the last ten seconds, the computer in

the last five, and communications satellites in the last second. The laser beam--perhaps the most potent medium of communication of all--appeared only a fraction of a second ago.

And they illustrate this with the field of medicine, too:

> ...in medicine, you would have almost no significant changes until about one minute ago. In fact, until one minute ago, as Jerome Frank has said, almost the whole history of medicine is the history of the placebo effect. About a minute ago, antibiotics arrived. About ten seconds ago, open-heart surgery. In fact, within the past ten seconds there probably have been more changes in medicine than is represented by all the rest of the time on our clock. (pp. 10-11)

This means that telemedicine, personalized genomics, digestible sensors, virtual dissection, wearable e-skins and evidence-based mobile health, to mention only a few, happened over the past two seconds.

This rapid change and bureaucracy are responsible for patient dissatisfaction, for malpractice suits, and for the erosion of doctor-patient communication. There is an essential mindlessness about medical bureaucracy which, as in other areas, causes it to accelerate entropy rather than to avoid it. As Postman and Weingartner explain, bureaucracies are the repositories of conventional assumptions and standard practices--two of the greatest accelerators of entropy. And this makes the subversive role of doctors, necessary. Subversive doctors are flexible, they know the difference between the word and the thing – between the book diagnosis and the specific patient, they are skillful in making distinctions between statements of fact, inferences and judgments, they are skilled in all important language behaviors such as asking meaningful questions; they are persistent in examining their own assumptions; they use definitions and metaphors as instruments for their thinking but are not trapped by them; they can move comfortably up and down the ladder of abstraction, depending on the patient and the context. And they are creative in unearthing other people's definitions and finding ways around them for the sake of their patients, as in Hassan's story.

The attitudes of the subversive doctor are reflected in her behavior. Her basic mode of discourse with patients is questioning and listening. She practices "Personalized Semantic Medicine" which means that her diagnoses stem from specific patients and their personal experience of illness, and not from an objective list of symptoms. And so do her prescriptions.

Subversive doctoring means treating the whole child. It means dealing not with the organ from which his illness stems, but with the child's body, his intellect, his emotions and his spirit. It means seeing each child as the individual that he is and not as part of a category such as "children with cerebral palsy." It means seeing that the child that Shelley was a few months ago on her previous visit, is not who she is now, in spite of the static nature of her name and of the word we use to call her disease or the combination of symptoms she displays, because things are always in a process of change – especially children. As Postman and Weingartner (1975) put it:

> It means understanding that even the phrase "the whole child" is as static a metaphor; that "child" is a thing word, a process transformed into a thing by our naming into a noun, and there is no stage of human growth that is more visibly a process than "childhood."
> (p. 172)

It means remembering, for example, that the word "psychosomatic" was coined to express a relationship and a process, explicitly to deter us from thinking that illness can always be categorized as either physical or mental. But that what happened eventually, is that we began to use it as a synonym for "mental," dismissing suffering as "merely psychosomatic."

Subversive doctors focus on the individuality and the uniqueness of every patient and abandon the assumption of sameness in all of them. They practice what is usually referred to as "patient-centered medicine" or "Personal Semantic Medicine" in our terms, keeping in mind that just as knowledge does not exist outside the learner, so disease does not exist outside the patient. They try to avoid projecting as much as possible, and not to transfer their own feelings and evaluations to their patients and their parents.

Aware that language is our most profound and possibly least visible environment, the subversive doctor remains constantly aware of the process of abstraction, and adopting an extensional approach, talks to her patients and encourages them to talk to her, in language that has accurate correspondence with externally verifiable meanings.

Subversive doctors keep a clean semantic environment. They insist on communicating with their patients in all the ways that are becoming less and less obvious to the culture; on having real and not only virtual relationships with their patients: providing clear information, involving patients in decision-making, following up consistently and educating patients on their conditions, all face-to-face and all resulting in improved physiologic as well as emotional health.

In short, subversive doctors are general semanticists. They are not fanatics. Fanaticism begins, as Postman (1976) explains, when we fall in love with certain sentences; when we internalize sentences to which we are so attached, that they are immune to criticism – others' and our own. The subversive physician is willing to permit the sentences to be scrutinized, subjected to criticism, and revised as their deficiencies require. He is aware of his fallibility and assumes that it is not possible for anyone to know if he or she is in possession of the "truth." This is important because the beliefs, feelings, and assumptions of doctors are the air of the medical environment; they determine the quality of life within it. If the air is polluted, the bronchitis may be cured, but the patient will have been poisoned and she will have contracted a new disease. When the air is polluted, the environment becomes useless, and, in Postman's words, it stops serving the purposes it is supposed to serve.

CONCLUSION

From Firearms to Paintbrushes:
Reviving the Metaphor of Medicine as Art

———■———

THE WORD "PANACEA" in the title of this book refers, of course, to the goddess of universal remedy in Greek mythology. Along with her sisters--the iatric graces--Panacea was the daughter of Asclepius, the demi-god of medicine and healing and of Epione, the goddess of soothing pain. Each one of her sisters performed a different facet of Apollo's art: Hygieia was the goddess of cleanliness, sanitation and the prevention of sickness; Iaso was the goddess of recuperation from illness; Aceso, the goddess of the healing process; and Aegle, the goddess of beauty, splendor, of radiant good health. And there were also four brothers, two of whom were also gods of medicine: Podaleirus, who had a flair for diagnostics, and Machaon, who was a master surgeon.

Panacea is perhaps the most famous of all of the iatric graces in modern times, as her name became a synonym for a universal remedy and it is used figuratively to describe something intended to completely solve a large, multi-faceted problem.

A word of clarification is in order here as it may seem as hubris on our part to suggest that efficient and effective communication is a universal remedy for all iatrogenic disease – certainly if at the basis of our theory are the central concepts of General Semantics, one of which is the idea that one can never say the last word on any matter; that a map does not represent all of a territory; that a word does not represent all of the "facts." To suggest that our remedy is universal would leave no room for "etc." – a reminder to be conscious of characteristics left out. However, it is our belief that effective communication has good potential of providing a comprehensive remedy or, better yet, a universal medication for the prevention of Semantic Iatrogenic Disease – for the iatrogenic ailments that result from physicians' misuses of language and their pollution of the medical semantic environment.

The importance of communication in the relationship between doctors and patients was understood as early as Hellenic medicine, as the understanding is reflected in the Hippocratic Oath--perhaps the most famous text in the history of medicine. The Oath articulates many of the central moral values that continue to guide medicine and that define what it means to be a medical professional to this day, among which are: privacy and confidentiality; the primacy of patients' welfare; a vow of chastity along with prohibition of sexual contact with or exploitation of patients; and prohibition of drugs for suicide.

Even though many doctors have taken the Oath, few of them over the centuries have actually cared much about the Greek gods and goddesses. But the Hippocratic Oath remains the historical loadstone for the professional values of privacy, confidentiality, and the promise to first and foremost, do no harm. And yet, some of its elements seem to have been forgotten or neglected with the passing of time, especially the one dealing with the importance of good communication with patients, represented most significantly by the demi-god Asclepius.

As is clear from the first line of the Oath, secular Hippocratic medicine did not set itself against the medicine of earlier gods of healing but rather appealed to them to sanctify its Oath.

> I swear by Apollo, the healer, Asclepius, Hygieia, and
> Panacea, and I take to witness all the gods, all the

goddesses, to keep according to my ability and my judgment, the following Oath and agreement...

Of all of the multiple gods of healing, only four are mentioned and, among them, Asclepius, whose greatness is said to be due, to a great extent, to his abilities as communicator. According to Hartigan (2009), Asclepios, Panacea's father, was not a god, but a demigod, a distinction that marks him as a terrestrial god. This ambiguity is reflected in his offspring. Each of his family members is a personification of an abstract iatric concept. His sons are always portrayed as mortals with good medical skills while his daughters are considered to share their father's divinity. Moreover, after his death, Asclepios did not rise to Mount Olympus. He remained on earth where his healing arts were needed. He was the prototype of the good doctor.

Unlike other gods, says Hartigan,

> ...he was always accessible and never really punished those who offended him. If someone failed to believe in his powers, he merely chided them, often by healing them as to disprove their doubt. He was a god who laughed at the foibles of mortals and from time to time teased them. When patients came to one of his sanctuaries, the statues they saw portrayed him as a kindly god...that seemed to invite mortals to approach him. (p. 24)

Perhaps it is the sense of humor, good communication skills and openness that explain why in the *Iliad,* Asclepios is called "the blameless physician."

As Marketos (1997) explains, ancient Hellenic medicine was based on the coexistence of both Asclepian (traditional) and

Hippocratic (rational) medicine. Both seem to have shared an ecological view of medicine from both the point of view of the geography or physical environment, and the human body and mind. First, the temples dedicated to Asclepios--called Asclepieia-- developed into therapeutic centers, where, besides his adoration, medical care was given by the priests. The locations for the establishment of the Asclepieia were selected taking into account the influence of climate and water supply to offer a naturally healthy environment to patients. And Hippocratic physicians are said to have treated the whole patient, not only the organs of the body.

Hippocratic medicine also took into account the semantic environment as is reflected in its sharing of human suffering and the idea that the place of a physician is at the bedside of his patient. When the Hippocratic physician went to the patient's home he had the duty to persuade not only the patient but the relatives, following the more communal character of life in antiquity. If he was called to undertake the treatment of a serious disease, he could refuse or accept, explaining the slight prospects of a cure. And in situations with a predictable fatal outcome, intervention was prohibited.

Furthermore, Hippocratic doctors had to possess the communication skills that make for a healthy semantic environment. As Marketos (1997) explains, the Hippocratic physician had to possess the oratorical skill to express his ideas about human nature and the structure and composition of the body as well as to answer the medical questions of the people, or simply for the better handling of human relations.

In his treatises, Hippocrates defined the ethical principles guiding medical practice. His entire work was inspired by humanistic ideals and a dedication to the patient. And he seems to have understood the idea of the context of the semantic environment generally, as well as of the power of what General Semantics calls "indexing." The healing art, according to Hippocrates, is linked to three conditions: the disease, the patient and the physician. Hippocrates believed that every patient was a different case and that this individuality made a fixed dogma for curative methods, impossible.

Nowadays, as previously mentioned, the Hippocratic bedside examination seems to have almost disappeared, pushed aside by modern technology. And doctors certainly don't go to patients' homes anymore. The perception of every patient as an autonomous person is made difficult by the idolatry of technology, by Evidence Based Medicine, by the rule of money and the 8-15 minute appointment standard. These have turned the clinic into an apparatus of bureaucratic administration applying principles and methods to whole categories of medical cases, dealing with sickness rather than with the sick. In spite of the fact that awareness of the logic of Personalized Genetic Medicine is rising, this applies mostly to the lab and less to the clinic, to the search for cures and not to the healing process or to doctoring. The need for "Personalized Semantic Medicine" is still less recognized. And patients themselves can play a key role in its advancement.

One of the iatrogenic illnesses afflicting most of us, is what Johnson (1946) called IFD disease. IFD stands for the process or progression from one state of mind to another--Idealization, Frustration and Demoralization--and it is a result of the use of words with vague referents in reality. For example, if along with calling the illness "cancer," doctors also connect their language with real and specific possibilities, they lead patients to the important goal of defining their expectations for themselves, specifically and realistically. This allows them to not encase themselves in what Johnson would call the "verbal cocoons" of the medical semantic environment in which doctors so often unreflectively employ the vague language that fosters frustration and demoralization.

It is possible that frustration and demoralization these days stem, at least in part, from the idealization of doctors and hospitals by the mass media. Assuming that the media generally and television specifically shape, at least to some degree, our conceptions of different aspects of life, it may be that *ER, Grey's Anatomy, House, Scrubs*, and other popular TV series, have created an image of doctors and of health care in our minds modelled after their characters whose charisma always stems not only from their professionalism but mostly from their kindness, empathy and gentle communication with patients.

As Turow (2010) explains, the people who work in television are much more concerned about the drama on medical shows than they are about the politics of medicine or changes in the medical system. And the gap between them leads to some tensions. Medical dramas have both exploited and shaped the audience's perceptions of medicine.

Regardless of whether people learn about specific conditions and procedures from watching these shows--a popular topic of discussion in television research--one thing seems quite clear: The shows usually represent an idealized view of doctors – the kind we would want looking after us when we are being hauled out of an ambulance. It is clear that almost all television indulges in dramatic license, for its own needs and reasons. But our point here is that as people find themselves grappling with reforms in their health-care systems, it can be frustrating and demoralizing for even the most critical viewer to experience an 8 minute visit with the doctor after spending 20 minutes filling out forms and waiting for another 20 to be called in, while being exposed on TV to doctors who seem to be able to spend all the money they want on extraordinary tests and procedures and all the time in the world on long conversations with patients. And they even make house calls.

These doctors are not always perfect. They are portrayed as fallible but always caring and with impeccable bedside manner. Even if they are arrogant at first, by the end of the episode we discover that deep inside they are good people. And most of what we see them doing is talking to patients.

Doctors have been at the center of innumerable stories since long before television. In literature there were, for example, Dr. Bernard Rieux in Camus's *The Plague*; Dorn in Chekhov's *The Seagull* or Astrov in his *Uncle Vanya*; Joseph Heller's Dr. "Doc" Daneeka in *Catch 22*; Dr. Heidegger in *Dr. Heidegger's Experiment* by Nathaniel Hawthorne, and Boris Pasternak's *Dr. Zhivago*. And in film, there were the deeply human Dr. Malcolm Sayer in *Awakenings* or Dr. Wilbur Larch in *The Cider House Rules*; to mention only a few.

It is only natural that writers and directors have chosen medicine and doctors as the basis for their stories, as these have the potential for fascinating human drama. But as opposed to Chekhov's doctors, for example, who struggle with depression and burnout, with incompetent co-workers and with their own flaws, and whose stories raise the big questions about the meaning and purpose of life and the manner it ought to be conducted, the doctors and hospitals on television are dream doctors and hospitals and they lead to their idealization. This is followed by frustration and demoralization when we meet our doctors in real life. As Brian Lowry suggested, in his column in *Variety* on June 26th, 2009, perhaps the Obama administration should enlist TV writers and the medical consultants that they employ to take the lead in revamping the health-care industry.

The solution to at least some of the ailments of health care may be found, of course, only if there's a change in the semantic environment of medicine as we encounter it in real life and not in that of any of its renditions in popular culture. Our focus throughout the book was placed on doctors as the professionals and authority figures chiefly in charge of the situation. But the change in the semantic environment is also partly in our hands – in the hands of patients who can immunize themselves against semantic iatrogenesis using the same tools available to physicians: an awareness of the semantic environment and the language we use in it. The remedy or communication panacea works best when as patients, we see ourselves as partners in the transaction and elicit from doctors the language and behavior that leads to the best cure for us.

In an age of what Postman (1992) calls "Information Glut," we have become credulous creatures, and this is especially true when it comes to issues pertaining to science or medicine framed in sentences that begin with the words "research shows." We have come to see physicians as magicians, we have reified illness and cures, and when the magicians fail to deliver the magic, we contract IFD in addition to what was originally ailing us. And then we sue doctors for malpractice.

Reification means confusing words with things and believing that things have real names. Our belief in real names originates in a kind of semantic illusion sometimes referred to as the principle of identity. And one of our deepest intuitions is to respond to the symbols we invent as if they are whatever it is that we invented them to symbolize.

Diagnoses are names doctors give to a host of different conditions, each of which manifest themselves and are handled differently by every one of us as patients. And yet doctors still call them the same, as if what we were experiencing were a thing – the same thing that others are experiencing. As was illustrated in Ami's story, when we speak of a child who "is" sick with an illness, we come to think of the child and the illness as inherently, immutably linked, forgetting that a definition is not a manifestation of nature but an instrument in the hands of our physicians, helping them achieve their purposes.

To reify words is to invest them with sacredness and therefore, to reverse the relationship that they may be assumed to have with "reality." As Postman (1976) explains, in some environments-- especially religious environments--the reversal is at the heart of the system. A wafer does not symbolize the body of Christ, it is the body; a cow for the Hindus is not a symbol of a sacred idea, it is the idea. And in the religion referred to as "medicine," we react to the word "cancer" for example, as if it were the illness.

Rather than act as obedient and adoring or awe struck parishioners, patients should try to strip away the sacredness attached to doctors, to diffuse any air of omnipotence around them, their diagnoses and their definitions, and so to avoid the devotion that ensues with the utterance of the word; they should ask questions and demand that the doctors bring their words down the ladder of abstraction, explain and elucidate them, speak them in the clearest way possible; if it is not inherently offered, they should ask for the comfort and listening that they need.

This is especially important in pediatrics. As the adults responsible for our children's wellbeing, we should remind doctors that, in the end, the whole family is the patient; that we are the main source of our children's psychological stability, and that we can be helpful in the diagnosis and treatment of all of our kids' problems, certainly when these are behavioral or psychosocial.

Patients should insist that doctors curb their skepticism. As Edwin Leap explains in his blog in *KevinMD.com* on March 18,

2014, skepticism and cynicism are important and useful. They make doctors look twice at a child's fracture and wonder if it was abuse and to question if a pharmaceutical company-sponsored study is truly useful. But we should insist that they be aware of their generalizations, look at us as individuals and remember we are not all drug-seekers or liars. Moreover, sometimes even drug seekers may have a ruptured aneurysm.

As patients, we should insist on communication so that we can cooperate with doctors and help them find that it wasn't a fall but abuse; that the source of our chest pain is our deep depression; that sometimes even those prone to anxiety attacks can get a pulmonary embolus; and that our child's stomach aches started when our cat died. We should insist on actively participating in the design of the medical semantic environment and working together with our doctors to find a new metaphor to replace the existing ones – whether it is the martial metaphors of general medicine discussed by Sontag (1988) or the veterinary metaphors of pediatrics as discussed by Gillis and Loughlan (2007).

Coulehan (2003) discusses the metaphor of medicine as war – where disease is the enemy, the doctor is the warrior captain and the patient is the battleground and Periyakoil (2008) illustrates the use of this metaphor with commonly used phrases such as "fighting a valiant battle with cancer," which creates an artificial win–lose dichotomy obligating the soldier-patient to fight to the end.

This is a problematic metaphor as it implies, for example, that opting to refuse futile or harmful treatment options, becomes equivalent to a cowardly retreat from the "battleground" that may be seen as a shameful act by the patient.

But these are not all of the metaphors that characterize the discourse and shape thought and action in medicine. The authors discuss additional metaphors such as sports metaphors. These invoke all the sports-related axioms and polarize outcomes as win or lose and they also perpetuate the myth that the patient and the illness are playing on opposing teams and that in order to be a true sportsman, the patient has to play it out until the end because quitting the game means loss of face.

There are also engineering metaphors that equate disease to malfunction, the physician to an engineer or a technician, and the patient to a machine with faulty parts that can be removed and replaced. And Coulehan (2003) also talks about parental metaphors in which disease is a threat or a danger, the physician is a loving parent, and the patient is a child – a metaphor fit for the treatment of children, but patronizing, infantilizing and dangerous in the care of adults.

When extended, there are, of course, faults to every metaphor. But we believe that the medical semantic environment may become a cleaner one if instead of being used as an empty cliché, the guiding metaphor becomes that of medicine as art.

The "art or science" debate about medicine has pervaded the literature in medicine for a very long time, sparked originally by the different, and yet complimentary, approaches of Asclepius and Hippocrates. Over the past few decades, there seems to be an agreement that medicine is both science and art, that the two views are complimentary. Those who are more specific talk about the practice of medicine as "art based on science."

However, whereas it is clear to all what makes medical research scientific, it is hard to find in the literature an explanation of what is meant by clinical medicine or the practice of medicine as an art.

What we suggest here is that clinical medicine be viewed not only as an art in the sense of an applied science, but that it take its place at the side of poetry, sculpture, drama and painting. This metaphor may slow down the decline in doctor-patient relationships, as what it implies is doctors as artists, patients as works of art, and diseases as the specific materials that individual patients are made of: canvas, paper, watercolors or oil, clay or bronze; tragedy or comedy, book, stage or screen. No two works of art are the same, and they each require a different approach, different moods and muses. Yet they are all the matter in the hands of artists at the service of the love of their art and their inspiration.

The communication panacea requires paintbrushes, not weapons. Not "fighting" illness--giving up the war metaphor--does not mean, in Ehrenreich's (2009) words, "greeting cancer with a smile." What it means is replacing this metaphor with a different one for thought and action in the process of coping with illness, and saving the analogy of war for what it is truly needed – our battle for the healthcare we deserve.

BIBLIOGRAPHY

———

Boisvert, C. W., Faust, D. (2002). Iatrogenic symptoms in psychotherapy: A theoretical exploration of the potential impact of labels, language, and belief systems. *Faculty Publications*, 41. Retrieved from http://digitalcommons.ric.edu/facultypublications/41

Cassell, E.J. (1985). *Talking with patients: The theory of doctor-patient communication* (Vol. 1). Cambridge, Mass: MIT Press.

Cassell, E.J. (1985). *The healer's art*. Cambridge, Mass: MIT Press.

Cassell, E.J. (1997). *Doctoring: The nature of primary care medicine*. Oxford, UK: Oxford University Press.

Canguilhem, G. (1989). *The normal and the pathological*. NY: Zone Books.

Castro, C.M., Wilson, C., Wang, F., & Schillinger, D. (2007, Sep/Oct). Babel Babble: Physician's use of unclarified medical jargon with patients. *American Journal of Health Behavior, Suppl.* 85-95.

Cegala, D. J., & Street, R. L., Jr. (2009). Interpersonal dimensions of health communication. In C. R. Berger, M. E. Roloff, & D. Roskos-Ewolsen (Eds.), *Handbook of Communication Science* (2nd Ed.) (pp. 401-417). Thousand Oaks, CA: Sage.

Charmaz, K. (2000). Experiencing chronic illness. In G. Albrecht, R. Fitzpatrick & S.C. Scrimshaw (Eds.), *Handbook of Social Studies and Health and Medicine* (pp. 277-292). London, UK: Sage.

Clandinin, D.J., & Caine, V. (2008). Narrative inquiry. In L. M. Given (Ed.), *The Sage Encyclopedia of Qualitative Research Methods* (pp. 541-544). Thousand Oaks, CA: Sage.

Connolly, C. (2005). Growth and Development of a Specialty: The Professionalization of Child Health Care. *Pediatric Nursing, 31*(3), 211-213, 215.

Coulehan, J. (2003). Metaphor and medicine: narrative in clinical practice. *Yale Journal of Biology and Medicine, 76*(2), 87–95.

Cushing, H. (1925, April). The life of Sir William Osler. *Bulletin of the Medical Libraries Association. 14*(4), 50.

Delvecchio Good, M.J, & Good, B. (2000). Clinical narratives and the study of contemporary doctor-patient relationships. In G. L. Albrecht, R. Fitzpatrick, & S. Scrimshaw (Eds.). *Handbook of Social Studies in Health and Medicine.* London, UK: Sage.

Ehrenreich, B. (2009). *Bright-Sided: How positive thinking is undermining America.* New York: Picador.

Ellul, J. (1964). *The technological society.* NY: Random House.

Emanuel, E.J., & Emanuel, L.L. (1992). Four models of the physician-patient relationship. *JAMA, 267* (16), 2221-2226.

Garrison, W.T., Bailey, E.N., Garb, J., Ecker, B., Spencer, P., & Sigelman, D. (1992). Interactions between parents and pediatric primary care physicians about children's mental health. *Hospital and Community Psychiatry, 43*(5), 489-493.

Gesell, A. (1940). *The first five years of life: A guide to the study of the preschool child, from the Yale Clinic of Child Development.* New York, NY: Harper and Brothers.

Gillis, J., Loughlan, P. (2007, Nov.). Not just small adults: the metaphors of paediatrics. *Archives of Disease in Childhood, 92*(11), 946–947.

Green, M., & Solnit, A.J. (1964). Reactions to the threatened loss of a child: A vulnerable child syndrome. *Pediatrics, 34*(1), 58-66.

Groopman, J. (2008). *How doctors think*. NY: Houghton Mifflin Company.

Hartigan, K. (2009). *Performance and cure: drama and healing in ancient Greece and contemporary America*. London: Duckworth Publishers

Hartzband, P., & Groopman, J. (2011, Oct.). The New Language of Medicine. *New England Journal of Medicine, 365*(15).

Hayakawa, S.I. (1963). *Symbol, Status, and Personality*. NY: Harcourt, Brace, Jovanovich.

Hilfiker, D. (1985). *Healing the wounds: A physician looks at his work*. NY: Pantheon Books.

Horwitz, S.M., Leaf, P.J., & Leventhal, J.M. (1998). Identification of psychosocial problems in pediatric primary care: Do family attitudes make a difference? *Archives of Pediatric and Adolescent Medicine, 152*(4), 367-371.

Illich, I. (1975). Clinical damage, medical monopoly, the expropriation of health: Three dimensions of iatrogenic tort. *Journal of Medical Ethics, 1*, 78-80

Illich, I. (1976). *Medical nemesis: The expropriation of health*. NY: Random House.

Johnson, W. (1946). *People in quandaries: The semantics of personal adjustment.* NY: Harper & Brothers.

Johnson, W. (1947, Apr.). How to ask questions. *Journal of General Education, 1*(2).

Keiger, D. (1998, Feb.). Why metaphors matter. *Johns Hopkins Magazine.*   Retrieved   from http://www.jhu.edu/~jhumag/0298web/metaphor.html

Kleinman, A., & Seeman, D. (2000). Personal experience of illness. In G. L. Albrecht, R. Fitzpatrick, & S. Scrimshaw (Eds.), *Handbook of Social Studies in Health and Medicine* (pp. 230-242). London, UK: Sage.

Korzybski, A. (1958). *Science and Sanity: An introduction to non-Aristotelian systems and General Semantics* (4th ed.). CT: Institute of General Semantics.

Laing, R.D., Phillipson, H., & Lee, A.R. (1966) *Interpersonal perception: a theory and a method of research.* London: Tavistock.

Lakoff, G., & Johnson, M. (1980). *Metaphors we live by.* Chicago, IL: University of Chicago Press.

Lee, I.J. (1994). *Language habits in human affairs* (2nd ed., S. Berman, Ed.). Concord, CA: International Society for General Semantics.

Leopold, N., Cooper, J., & Clancy, C. (1996). Sustained partnership in primary care. *Journal of Family Practice, 42*(2), 129-137.

Levinson, W. (1997, Mar.). Doctor-Patient communication and medical malpractice: Implications for pediatricians. *Pediatric Annals*, *26*(3), 186-193.

Marketos, S.G. (1997). The parallels between Asclepian and Hippocratic medicine on the island of Kos. *American Journal of Nephrology*, *17*, 205–208.

Peabody, F. (1927, Mar.). The Care of the Patient. *The Journal of the American Medical Association.* *8*(12), 882.

Periyakoil, V. (2008). Using Metaphors in Medicine. *Journal of Palliative Medicine*, *11*(6).

Pollio, H., Graves, T. R., & Arfken, M. (2006). Qualitative methods. In F. T. L. Leong & J. T. Austin (Eds.), *The psychology research handbook* (2nd ed.) (pp. 254-274). Thousand Oaks, CA: Sage.

Postman, N. (1969). Demeaning of meaning. In N. Postman, C. Weingartner & T. Moran. *Language in America: A report on our deteriorating semantic environment.* NY: Pegasus (pp.13-20).

Postman, N. (1976). *Crazy Talk, Stupid Talk: How we defeat ourselves by the way we talk and what to do about it.* New York: Dell Publishing Co., Inc.
Postman, N. (1982). *The Disappearance of Childhood.* NY: Dell.

Postman, N. (1992). *Technopoly: The surrender of culture to technology.* NY: Alfred Knopf.

Postman, N., & Weingartner, C., (1969). *Teaching as a Subversive Activity.* NY: Delacorte Press.

Postman, N., & Weingartner, C., (1975, August, 1). Thingness. *Pediatrics*, 56(2).

Reiser, S.J., (1978). *Medicine and the reign of technology*. MA: Cambridge University Press.

Shaw, G. B. (1911). *The Doctor's Dilemma*. NY: The Trow Press.

Shorter, E. (1991). *Doctors and Their Patients: A Social History*. New Brunswick, NJ: Transaction Books.

Sontag, S. (1988). *Illness as metaphor*. NY: Farrar, Straus, Giroux

Sontag, S. (1989). *AIDS and its metaphors*. NY: Farrar, Straus & Giroux.

Spock, B. (2004). *Baby and child care* (8th ed.). NY: Gallery Books.

Strate, L.(2008). Studying media as media: McLuhan and the Media Ecology approach. *MediaTropes eJournal*, *1*, 127–142.

Strate, L. (2011). *On the binding biases of time and other essays on general semantics and media ecology*. TX: The New Non Aristotelian Library, Institute of General Semantics.

Streisand, R., & Tercyak, K. (2004). Parenting chronically ill children: The scope and impact of Pediatric Parenting Stress. In M. Hoghughi & N. Long (Eds.) *Handbook of parenting: Theory and research for practice* (pp. 181-197). London, UK: Sage.

Taleb, N.N. (2012). *Antifragile: Things that gain from disorder*. NY: Random House.

Turow, J. (2010). *Playing Doctor: Television, Storytelling, and Medical Power*. Ann Arbor, MI: University of Michigan Press.

Wallander, J.L., Varni, J.W., Babani, L., Banis, H.T., & Wilcox, K.T. (1989). Family resources as resistance factors for psychological maladjustment in chronically ill and handicapped children. *Journal of Pediatric Psychology, 14* (2), 157-173.

Wildavsky, A. (1977, Winter). Doing better and feeling worse: The political pathology of health policy. *Daedalus 106*(1), 105.

Williams, W. C. (1984). *The doctor stories*. New York, NY: New Directions.

INDEX

EVA BERGER is a Professor of Communication at the School of Media Studies of COMAS (College of Management Academic Studies) in Israel where she was Dean (2006-2012). Dr. Berger is member of the Board of Trustees of the Institute of General Semantics (since 2009) and of *ETC.: A Review of General Semantics* (since 2008). She is member of the Editorial Board of *Giluy Daat: A Multidisciplinary Journal on Education, Society and Culture* (since 2011) and was member of the Editorial Board of *EME: Explorations in Media Ecology* (2005-2014). She has held many public positions and is active in numerous organizations in Israel: She was member of the search committee for candidates for the position of Chair of the Council for Cable and Satellite Communications (appointed in 2013 by the Minister of Communication); Chair of the Board of *Women in the Picture* (an organization for the advancement of women in the visual arts); member of the Israel Press Council (2011-2013) and of the Israeli Film Board (2000-2006). She is member of the board of IPI (Israel Peace Initiative, since 2011). Eva is periodically invited as guest commentator on Israel's newspapers and public and private radio and television stations; she is the author of programs for the teaching of media in Israel's high schools; and has published numerous academic articles and book chapters on varying topics including war photojournalism; advertising; language, metaphor and narrative; and media and technology. Eva is married and has two sons.

ISAAC BERGER studied medicine at UNAM--National University of Mexico in Mexico City (1955-1961). He did his internship as well as his residency in Pediatrics at Michael Reese Hospital in Chicago and was research fellow in neonatology there. In 1965, he returned to his country of origin—Mexico—where along with his private practice throughout the years, he was instructor of postgraduate courses in Pediatrics at Juarez Hospital; assistant lecturer in Pediatrics at UNAM (National University of Mexico); lecturer in Pediatrics at the School of Nursing as well as at the residency program of American British Cowdray Hospital in Mexico City; and he taught neonatology at Hospital Infantil Privado where he was physician in charge of Medical Education. In 1977 Dr. Berger moved with his family to Israel where he became Head of the Pediatric Outpatient Department of Meir General Hospital in the city of Kfar Saba, and later Head of Pediatric Ambulatory Services (including Emergency Room, Clinics, Day Hospital Unit, and Child Development Unit). Isaac co-authored numerous articles and chapters in books. He retired from the hospital in 2003 and aside from his still active private practice he is medical advisor to a large child development center in Israel. Isaac is married and has five daughters and nine grandchildren.

CPSIA information can be obtained
at www.ICGtesting.com
Printed in the USA
JSHW050102250822
29636JS00001B/97